HOW TO EAT RIGHT & SAVE THE PLANET

A PLANT-BASED SURVIVAL GUIDE
FOR YOU & YOUR FAMILY

BILL TARA

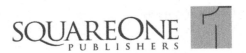

SQUAREONE
PUBLISHERS

The information and advice contained in this book are based upon the research and the personal and professional experiences of the author. They are not intended as a substitute for consulting with a health care professional. The publisher and author are not responsible for any adverse effects or consequences resulting from the use of any of the suggestions, preparations, or procedures discussed in this book. All matters pertaining to your physical health should be supervised by a health care professional. It is a sign of wisdom, not cowardice, to seek a second or third opinion.

COVER DESIGNER: Jeannie Rosado
IN-HOUSE EDITOR: Erica Shur
TYPESETTER: Gary A. Rosenberg

Square One Publishers
115 Herricks Road
Garden City Park, NY 11040
(516) 535-2010 • (877) 900-BOOK
www.squareonepublishers.com

Library of Congress Cataloging-in-Publication Data
Names: Tara, Bill, author.
Title: How to eat right & save the planet : a plant-based survival guide
    for you and your family / Bill Tara.
Description: Garden City Park, NY : Square One Publishers, [2020] |
    "Spotting the food fantasies that are destroying our health." |
    Includes bibliographical references and index.
Identifiers: LCCN 2019019255 (print) | LCCN 2019022372 (ebook) | ISBN
    9780757004865 (paperback : alk. paper)
Subjects: LCSH: Vegetarianism—Health aspects. | Natural foods—Health
    aspects. | Environmental health.
Classification: LCC RM236 .T37 2019 (print) | LCC RM236 (ebook) | DDC
    613.2/62—dc23
LC record available at https://lccn.loc.gov/2019019255
LC ebook record available at https://lccn.loc.gov/2019022372

Printed in the United States of America

10   9   8   7   6   5   4   3   2

Contents

PART FOUR The Road Ahead

Acknowledgments

We are often unaware of those who inspire us when we first connect with them either in person or through their words or acts. Some stand out for me especially, my father Lyle (Bud) Tara was more at home in nature than under a roof. It made no difference if "The Captain" was in the wheelhouse at sea or in a deep forest, he was watchful and aware. He always said when leaving a camping site, "leave it like no one was here." He would have never called himself an environmentalist but that spirit was in his heart.

I was drawn to pick up the *Silent Spring* while in a book shop the year it came out and have been an enthusiastic supporter of Rachel Carson's work since then. She is a great example of the clear-eyed "science with a soul" that is most needed in these times. She was hounded to her death by corporate thugs and always a brave advocate for the living world.

Michio and Aveline Kushi and Shizuko Yamamoto were my introduction to Japanese culture and tradition. Michio was my mentor for many years and set me on a path to my life's work. He was tireless in his work to introduce the concepts of Japanese folk medicine and the Macrobiotic philosophy to the world. He and his wife Aveline were principle driving forces in the revolution that introduced natural, organic foods to the western world.

Over five decades there have been medical mavericks who have pushed back against the commercial influences in modern medicine and nutrition. Dr Robert Mendelson inspired me with his quick wit and unbending vision of a better kind of medicine. Drs Michael Klaper, Neil

Barnard, Professor T Colin Campbell, and John McDougall have always been at the forefront of the wave of new science that drives the move toward a healthy and earth friendly way of eating.

Professors Gary Francione and Anna Charlton are not only inspiring but also simply great people to be around. They have presented the moral and legal issues of veganism with outstanding clarity. Their willingness to stand against the hypocrisy of many "animal rights" groups displays the true spirit of social justice for human and non-human life.

My thanks to Emily Lamberty who kicked things off with some early research and Mary Murphy who did an early edit and critique. My thanks also go out to Rudy Shur of Square One for giving me the opportunity to get my book out into the world and to Erica Shur for editing my sometimes ragged prose. Students are always a good source of inspiration, those at the IMP in Lisbon, Portugal, always have good questions that keep me on my toes.

My old friend Francisco Varatojo was an easy listener and a sharp intellect and comrade of the soul. Our many conversations revolved around the issues contained here—he is much missed.

Lastly (certainly not least) my friend, my love, my Scottish muse, my wife Marlene, who has shared my every thought and supports me with affection, inspiration, and delicious healthy food on a daily basis.

Foreword

There are *many* books that talk about diet, health, and nutrition. There are, however, at least three reasons to read *How to Eat Right and Save the Planet* by Bill Tara.

The first reason is that Bill Tara, unlike many of the authors of other books on nutrition and health, is not a recent arrival on the scene. Bill was one of *the* founders of the natural health movement going back to the 1960s.

He was the Vice President of Erewhon Trading Company, one of America's first national distributors of organic foods, and was a co-founder of Sunwheel Natural Foods in London, England. He has been a health counsellor, teacher, author, entrepreneur, and creator of health education centers in Europe and North America.

In 1975 he founded the Community Health Foundation in London, England, a Charitable Trust that was the largest natural health education center in the world. Together with Michio and Aveline Kushi, who introduced macrobiotics to the West in the early 1950s, he was a founder of the Kushi Institute and served as Executive Director of the institute programs in London, England and Boston, USA. Bill has served as a senior faculty member at the Kiental Institute, an international macrobiotic educational center, in Switzerland, and the Naropa University in Boulder, Colorado. He was Chairman of the European Macrobiotic Assembly for four years and served as Chairman of the North American Macrobiotic Congress for two years.

His innovative and creative teaching of traditional approaches to health, healing, and personal development has taken him to over twenty countries as a lecturer. He has appeared on a variety of radio and television shows in England, America, and Australia speaking on health, diet, and the environment, including *Nightline* with Ted Koppel.

In 1975 he edited and published, *Your Face Never Lies,* based on the teachings of Michio Kushi, which continues to be one of the most popular books on Oriental diagnosis. In 1985 he published *Macrobiotics and Human Behaviour,* the first book by a Western writer on the Chinese theory of the body/mind connection. His latest published books include *Natural Body/Natural Mind,* a clarion call to us to make our lives whole again.

Bill and his partner, Marlene Watson-Tara, who is herself an expert in Chinese medicine and Oriental diagnosis, have created the Macrobiotic Vegan Health Coach Program, which has thus far brought students from 27 countries who have come to study with them and to train to become health counselors. Bill and Marlene also facilitate and run seminars and health retreats in various parts of Europe and America for private corporations. Their public programs and workshops are vast. They cover diet and the development of disease, social justice, food slavery, environmental issues, animal rights and more as part of their progressive vision of the Human Ecology Project.

That is a mere fraction of what one could say about Bill Tara. The point is that this book comes from a pioneer—a leader—of the natural health movement. He helped to introduce macrobiotics to the West. With Marlene, he has brought Chinese medicine and Oriental diagnosis to tens of thousands of people. This is a book of wisdom and perspective developed over a half century.

Second, this is not just a book about health and diet. It is a book that presents a *philosophy* that ties together diet and nutrition, health, ecology, animal rights, and social justice. I am well aware of what's out there and I can say that there is *nothing* else available that is remotely like this book. Bill presents an intelligent and progressive theory of human ecology. That said, the book is packed full with very practical advice on how to keep from getting ill and dying as a result of all the poison that we are told is "food." This book could very well save your life not only in terms of your body, but also in terms of your spirit.

Third, the book is sound, accessible, and thoroughly engaging. You won't want to put it down. And by the time you finish, you will be well on the way to a healthier mind and spirit, and you will be equipped and motivated to want to do your part to make a healthier and more just planet.

This book is one of the few books that you will come across that will truly change your life. I urge you to read it. I assure you that you will be grateful that you did.

Gary L. Francione
Board of Governors Distinguished Professor of
Law, and Nicholas deB. Katzenbach Scholar
of Law and Philosophy, Rutgers University

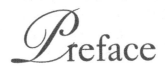

Preface

The very real crisis created by our food choices needs resolution and needs it quickly. The research has been done and the positive steps to a healthy diet have been identified, and yet the powerful machine that governs the food system grinds on with little sign of significant change. One fact is stunningly apparent: the modern diet is killing us and we are not acting to make the changes necessary. Part of the problem is that nutrition is not simply an issue of the chemical features of our foods. Cultural and emotional factors often seem to outweigh logic and ethics.

A modern vision of nutrition needs to take into account the social and environmental costs of what we eat as well as the price we pay at the market. Vested interests are so deeply embedded in the political, medical, agricultural, and food manufacturing sectors that powerful forces can be called into play when challenges are made to the status quo.

The internet has provided a perfect growing medium for fanciful nutritional theories, magical supplements, and direct attacks on any ideas that challenge cultural dietary traditions. There is no greater battlefield in the nutrition wars than the entrenched ideas we have about the use of animal sourced foods. It is time for a new understanding of our historical relationship to what we eat.

From our ancient origins, human life has migrated to almost every location on the planet. We have settled in deep jungles, arctic tundra, deserts, and forests. Our primary concern has always been to find food. It is a matter of life or death. We did not have to concern ourselves with eating locally or in season; that was a given. We ate what was available. The forces of nature were in charge.

If there was an abundance of nutritious plants, that was where we focused; if not, we used animals. We discovered over time that out of the 391,000 species of plants there are a fairly small number that are safe for us to eat and we focused on those. These were not decisions we made in a conference hall. Decisions were made through human experience. They were pragmatic actions aimed at staying alive and creating homeostasis, that life-producing relationship with nature that governs all life. That was then, this is now.

Nature is still in control. It is nature that supplies our air, water, and food—a simple truth we seem to have forgotten. When we look at the modern food chain, we see that we have made every attempt to break down that relationship. This is a futile and childish struggle to dominate rather than adapt and it has produced chaos. This struggle between humankind and nature lies at the root of much of the confusion and endless arguments about nutrition as well as ecology.

The modern diet produces disease and death, not only for humans but non-humans as well. Our food choices are the main cause of death from degenerative disease, creates environmental chaos, the senseless slaughter of billions of sentient creatures, and supports an economic system that makes regional self-sufficiency and food security impossible. Yet we march on. We fixate on fantasy stories about magical properties of the newest "super-food," the power of reducing the sugar content in soft drinks or avoiding meat one day a week. None of these stop-gap measures are effective or timely.

There is still time for us to make the easiest and most important contribution we can to creating a healthy world for all life on planet Earth. It is important that a new conversation about the food we eat is engaged in and that action is taken. We can change what we eat, right now, today and then move to more complicated issues.

$\mathscr{I}$ntroduction

There are powerful mythologies that drive our understanding of the foods we eat. Our knowledge of nutrition is not simply an issue of understanding the chemical structure of food, it is influenced by our culture, senses, emotion, economy, and environment. Our understanding into how these issues blend and affect each other has been slowly growing over the past decades. It has not been a smooth journey and it is not over.

The revolution in nutrition has been driven by laboratory scientists, epidemiological analysts, grass roots activists, environmentalists, and moral philosophers. This dedicated band has been engaged with the powerful forces of political lobbyists with multi-million dollar gifts to dispense, food industry giants who buy "scientific" research, and a medical brotherhood often locked in its own self-interests. If all this reminds you of the battles for the truth about the dangers of smoking or climate change, it should. It is the same game and it is killing us. The issue is simple: our modern diet not only creates disease, it endangers all life on the planet—and yes, that includes us.

Scientists are uncertain how many animals inhabit planet Earth. According to a recent study published in the journal *PLoS Biology*, there are 8.7 million species of animal life on our planet—and every year, new species are discovered. Every one of these species knows intuitively what to eat—except one. Only one creature knowingly and stubbornly eats food that causes it to get sick. Guess which?

The grim paradox is that the more information we have about what to eat, the more we seem to be confused. We are exposed to a daily tide of opinion, science, and advertising about what to eat, much of which is contradictory.

Partly in response to the growing epidemic of obesity, diet has become an emotional and controversial subject. A report from the US Food and Drug Administration states that Americans spend an estimated $40 billion a year on weight loss related products and health-related food, beverages, and services. Around 180 million people—*that's more than half our population*—are on a weight-loss diet at any given time and most of them will try four diets a year. Weight loss is big business.

I was raised in slightly less complicated times. Like most people, I never thought much about food unless I was hungry. There were certain foods I liked and others I didn't. When I was hungry, I ate—and sometimes I ate when I wasn't hungry. Sometimes I ate out of boredom and sometimes it was because there was something tasty close at hand. That all changed for me in the sixties. When I was twenty-four years old, I was a devoted hippie living in San Francisco, and the Summer of Love was just around the corner.

My roommate came home one day and told me he had just been "turned on" to a great book by a Japanese philosopher. The book explained how you could cure diseases and improve your consciousness at the same time by eating a special diet. He wanted to give it a try since he suffered from asthma. Our shared interest in Eastern philosophy and our "try anything one time" attitude launched us both in an unexpected direction.

We searched for the foods listed in the book and entered new territory. We started eating whole grains, beans, vegetables, and a variety of Japanese condiments. It was a 360-degree change. We discovered that there was a small but growing army of folks who were giving this a try. There were even some famous teachers right in the USA. After a rocky start—having to eat our mistakes—we got into the rhythm of our new way of eating.

The results, for me, were unexpected and impressive. Without even trying, I started to lose excess weight and to feel more energetic than I had in years. But the big bonus was not the size of my stomach but what was happening inside it.

Two years previously, the pains that I often experienced after eating started to intensify, until I finally went to see a doctor. Tests revealed that I had advanced ulceration in both stomach and duodenum—the passageway between the stomach and the small intestine. I was shocked and a little frightened. I associated ulcers with stressed-out middle-aged businessmen, not healthy young hippies. The doctor's assessment was that I must be living a stressful life and needed to relax. I was told that if the ulcers didn't get better, surgery was a possible alternative. Now I had a real reason to be stressed!

I was advised to use Pepto-Bismol to ease the symptoms. I was also given a prescription for some drugs and antacids, a slap on the back, and sent away with a diet sheet. The diet sheet suggested that I avoid all fibrous vegetables, roughage, and spicy foods, and to eat plenty of soft foods and drink milk. Aside from that, I was to eat a "balanced and healthy diet." In other words, I should continue eating the standard American diet with more Jell-O and baby food. For two years, none of that had made any difference. In fact, the ulceration got worse.

However, according to my new Japanese health plan, the medication and all drugs were off the table. The milk and any dairy food, meat, sugar, and processed foods were gone as well. My diet was filled with the dreaded roughage I had been warned against.

The results were obvious. Within weeks, I had no pain after eating or at any other time. I was sleeping well, and I felt wonderful. After a few months of eating this way, I decided to go back and have another round of tests. I returned to the doctor a week later for my results with a smile on my face and a typed copy of my diet plan in my pocket. I knew the ulcers were gone.

I had a bantering relationship with my doctor. She would tease me about being a hippie, and I would tease her about being "square." She said that the x-rays showed dramatic healing. The ulcers were on the run. The drugs had worked! She was thrilled—but not for long.

In my naiveté, I thought my doctor would be impressed. I knew there were improvements before the tests were back. I thought she would welcome sharing my diet discovery. After all, my cure was cheap, simple, and effective. All I did was to remove all meat, dairy, processed food, and sugar from my diet. How many people could be helped with this simple approach? There must be a Nobel Prize in there for someone.

I told her I hadn't taken the drugs for many months and gave her the diet I was on. To my surprise, she became quietly furious. After scanning the diet pages, she looked me square in the eye and told me through clenched teeth that it was all voodoo. She actually tore up the sheets and said that I would be back pleading with her to do surgery when my ulcers returned, and that I was no longer her patient if I insisted on following this crazy diet. I didn't know what to say except goodbye. I was dumbfounded and filled with questions.

The first of these questions was "Why the animosity?" The fact that the ulcers had healed was shown by objective medical criteria as well as my personal experience. This should at least have stimulated curiosity. She should have been happy. But her response was neither scientific nor logical; it was emotional.

The second question had to do with the origin of the information in the little book. "Why was this approach to health and diet, based on a system that was thousands of years old, more effective than modern science?" How did those ancient sages discover something that modern scientists missed? What did they know that we didn't? I was inspired to find answers to these questions,

I have spent the decades since that meeting searching out the answers to those two questions from sources in ancient wisdom and modern science, both the beliefs and the practices. I am thankful for the doctor's reaction. It sent me off in a direction I would have never expected. That search has led me to farmers and surgeons, food producers and philosophers, mystics and scientists. You will find what I discovered in the following chapters, which are divided into four parts.

Part One is comprised of Chapters One through Five. It begins by looking at "How Did We Get Here." How did refrigeration, supermarkets, chemical additives, and big business contribute to a false narrative on what healthy food was? To answer the question, this section addresses the poor choices of sugar, meat, and dairy for good nutrition and good health. It then shows how medicine and nutrition inhibited the preventive potential of nutrition but created a bogus "war on disease" in the process. It goes on to discuss how a revolution in health care and nutrition was driven by women, hippies, and a few brave doctors' intent on creating a new paradigm of health.

Part Two examines a different outlook on nutrition, "A Natural Perspective." Chapters Six, Seven, and Eight take us into the understanding of diet and health that is often referred to as "Traditional Medicine" and the intriguing possibility that what we eat influences what we think. These are the systems of folk medicine that represent centuries of experience, reflection, record keeping, and shared knowledge. I use the medicine of the Far East and the example of modern macrobiotics to illustrate how these approaches to health can help create a more effective approach to nutrition. All of those systems were ecological in their approaches. They respected the laws of nature and sought to create balance with them.

Part Three offers the big view of nutrition, its "Cause and Effect." Chapters Nine, Ten, and Eleven show how the modern diet produces consequences that ripple out into the world, often with devastating effects. These influences include deforestation as well as the degradation of the soil, water, and air quality. As you will come to understand in this section, this damage is reflected in human suffering as well. The modern diet not only causes disease but also a socially unjust system of food distribution. Food slavery and worker exploitation are essential to the modern food industry, it cannot exist without them. This section ends with a discussion on the ethical issues of animal use and the implications of our culture.

In Part Four's "The Road Ahead," Chapters Twelve, Thirteen, and Fourteen help you get started on the path to eating right. This section gives a detailed outline of what I call the *Human Ecology Diet*—a diet based on macrobiotic principles and the newest discoveries in nutritional science, ecological concerns, and vegan ethics. You will find a listing of the foods, vitamins, and minerals that have the highest potential in creating a healthy and sustainable plant-based diet and a survey of the nutritional benefits of those foods. The last chapter provides a few new life skills that are necessary if you pursue the *Human Ecology Diet* and to help create a healthy lifestyle.

This book is about connecting the dots between these diverse issues. It is also about providing solutions. Yes, there are answers to these problems, and the answers have been around for many years. Many brave men and women have highlighted the dangers of our attitudes to health and to the foods we eat. What we need is a shift in our thinking as well as in the foods we purchase, prepare, and consume. The problem is not a lack of information, but a lack of action. By the end of this book, I hope you come to understand that you can not only create health for yourself and your family, but you can also contribute to a healthy world for all life on planet Earth.

By the way, my friend cured his asthma.

PART ONE

How Did We Get Here?

I

$\mathcal{W}$ho's in the Kitchen?

We know that our food has changed over the centuries. Ever since the agricultural revolution 10,000 years ago our relationship with the production and processing of food has been transforming and with it we have changed nature. We cleared forests, claimed grassland, and generally placed our distinct foot print on the face of the planet. Along with the changes in agriculture have come changes in the nutritional substance of what we eat and how we feel about our food.

Much of what we eat today would be completely foreign to our grandparents. That change is a reflection of many factors. The way we grow our food, the techniques we use to process it, the systems we use to transport it, advertise it, and sell it have all gone through a massive transformation. We also know something else. The food in the market stores and in the fast food outlets and the snacks and treats we see advertised on TV are killing us. And I do mean *killing* us.

The food industry will claim that these changes improved the quality of what we eat, offer longer shelf-life, and will provide us with a new era of abundant food. We are even told that it is the healthiest diet in history. As we will see, all of those statements are false and shift attention away from the price we pay in terms of public health, social justice, and environmental damage. The reasons we continue to eat the products of this bloated and corrupt industry and even feed it to our children are many.

The issues of what we eat are not only limited to the industry that produces the food but also to personal habits, medical short-sightedness, political cowardice, and imagined traditions. To see through the smoke and mirrors, I want to start in the kitchen. As you may remember, that is the room where food was stored, prepared, and for so many centuries eaten.

I am going to focus on one particular period of the recent past: the years immediately before and following World War Two. It was a time when we experienced the greatest change in our food and in our relationship to what we eat.

HOME COOKING

Prior to the late 1940s, cooking generally happened at home. We knew where our food came from and who selected and cooked it. We were in control of what we ate. Usually it was a family member who prepared the family meal, most likely a mother or grandmother. Some of that food might have been from a family garden or a local provider. All that changed very rapidly within a single decade. I experienced these changes through my grandmother and my mother.

My mother, my sister, and I lived with my grandparents until I was ten. Grandma was the guardian of the kitchen. No one else was allowed to cook, not even the daughters or aunts. They might be summoned to assist, but Grandma was always in charge.

Going to the store with my grandmother was a challenge. She needed to know where everything came from; she smelled and poked, squeezed, and inspected every item. Carrots and apples, chickens, and greens—she knew what she was looking for and never settled for less. The shopkeepers were on high-alert when she showed up. The only packaged foods in our kitchen were baking supplies, sugar, and a few condiments. Everything was made from "scratch." Breads, cakes, stews, soups, mayonnaise, even ice cream—everything that came out of that kitchen was made there.

The kitchen changed with the seasons. The tail end of summer was the time of most intensive action. There were trips to the countryside to get boxes of fresh fruits and vegetables from farm stands. A canning operation was set up in the kitchen and on the back porch. We boiled large tubs of water to sterilize glass bell jars for dill pickles, succotash, sauerkraut, and endless jars of fruit and fruit preserves. The shelves in the garage were stocked with a colourful range of food to use during the winter. My grandmother loved cooking. It was a full-time commitment.

Things changed when I was eleven. My mother remarried, and we moved into a new home and had a new way of eating. Both my father and mother worked, time for food preparation was limited. I know she believed that she was giving us good food but some of the rules had changed. The folk traditions that had ruled the kitchen were being replaced by advertising and more processed foods. The marketplace was also being transformed. By the mid-1950s, Mom was faced with a new way of shopping and a growing abundance of new food products. The supermarket had moved into town.

I remember walking down those neon-lit aisles with yards of brightly packaged foods, refrigerated cases packed with meats and frozen products. It was like science fiction—so shiny, so antiseptic. Even the fruits and vegetables looked polished and pristine.

The food industry was devoted to helping Mom out of her pesky time problem. New cookbooks showed homemakers how to use condensed soups, packaged sauces, and cheap cuts of meat to add "variety" to the table. Frozen foods, with a quick cooking time, made seasonal vegetables available all year round. Betty Crocker promised you could make a cake in 5 minutes, Swanson foods promised a complete dinner in 25 minutes, what could be better?

THE COLD TRUTH

The generation that had grown up during the Great Depression and endured the Second World War wanted an easier life. Food became a primary commercial focus in this quest. Why spend time preparing food that could be purchased ready-made? Why wait an hour for dinner when it could be served piping hot in minutes? The two-income household was on the rise, and the growing middle class wanted everything to be more "streamlined," "modern," and "convenient." Corporate America used the desire for an easy life to sell easy-to-prepare food regardless of the health effects. Industry had taken over the nation's kitchens.

In the 1920s, the Birdseye Company had developed the flash-freezing process, enabling producers to deliver seafood and some vegetables without significant loss of taste. However, most small shops lacked the equipment to keep foods frozen, and many homes did not have refrigerators with freezing compartments. Appliance makers manufactured new refrigerators with large freezing compartments that became symbols of status in the modern home. By the late 1930s, the popularity of home refrigerators was growing; and after the Second World War, they became commonplace. By 1950, more than 90 percent of urban homes had refrigerators. These appliances increasingly contained larger freezer compartments. Supermarkets quickly expanded their refrigeration and could sell everything the family needed in one location. "One-stop" food shopping was born.

Refrigeration largely erased the problem of distance between food sources and consumers. Previously foods, such as fish, were difficult for consumers living far from the coasts to purchase, and most dairy foods, especially butter would not be possible to store without refrigeration. Now meat could be slaughtered at a great distance and with industrial speed and stored for months and shipped long distances without spoilage. It also meant that producers could hold food for very long times before releasing them to the market place. The "freshness factor" and its inherent effect on nutrition was undermined.

As a side note, our love affair with refrigeration was a very risky one. The early appliances used refrigerants like sulphur dioxide and methyl chloride; these toxic fumes were causing people to die. Ammonia was also used with similar effect. Without really exploring the downside of the chemicals used as refrigerants, we eventually would create massive damage to the ozone layer of the atmosphere. Chlorofluorocarbons (CHFs) and hydrochlorofluorocarbons (HCFCs) eventually depleted the ozone layer and needed to be outlawed in 1987.

With refrigeration, local and regional farming began a slow slide into oblivion. Seasonal eating went out the window. Regional and local farming were forced into a corner and could not compete with crops grown cheaply at a distant location and shipped long-distance out of season.

The supermarkets, coupled with proliferating fast-food outlets, were the most dramatic first steps toward the modern diet. By the late 1950s, both had become symbolic of American food culture. They also became international symbols of affluence and social privilege. The general public was thrilled by this "modern" quick, easy, and inexpensive food. Very few saw that there were hidden costs in these food products that would have to be paid later. Some of these costs were physical, some were environmental. Less obvious costs concerned how we perceived the value of food in our lives.

In our collective innocence, we assumed that the companies that made our food had our best interests in mind. Our food was no longer cooked; it was manufactured. Aside from the label, we often had no way of judging food quality. The food was canned, bottled, or otherwise concealed. Words like "natural," "nutritious," "healthy," or "wholesome" lost all meaning outside of advertising. A chasm was created between our food and ourselves.

The food industry already knew it was easy to make food look good and even taste fresher through the use of chemical additives and mechanical processing. Peas that turned gray in processing could be dyed a bright green. Unsellable tomatoes could be made into catsup and sauces, re-colored, re-flavored, and artificially thickened. Our manufactured food became a chemistry project.

As long as the product had a long shelf life, looked good, and had an acceptable taste, it was a winner. Oh, and predictability was a plus. A Swanson TV dinner was exactly the same in New York or Hawaii. As McDonald's was to discover, the consumer loves predictable.

The new supermarkets could store stock for longer periods of time. Assurances of "freshness" were impossible to verify. More chemical additives and preservatives gave us a diet with plenty of taste but not much flavor. This was a feast filled with chemicals and calories but with diminished nutritional value.

One of the results of eating pre-packaged foods is a reduction in the nutritional density of the foods consumed. This particularly affects children. It is an everyday nutritional deficiency experienced as more and more meals are ready-to-eat, fast foods are brought home to eat. One study showed that half the food energy that children consumed was from fast foods eaten in the home.

The Organization for Economic Cooperation and Development sponsored a study that showed that Americans spent an average of only thirty minutes a day on food preparation as compared to fifty-two minutes in other countries, and about 25 percent less time eating. We have given away the kitchen and now have no idea what's in the food we eat; it has been cleverly disguised.

THE CHEMISTRY PROJECT

The use of food additives and processing to assure preservation is not new. For thousands of years people smoked and dried meats, and they fermented a wide range of foods, from vegetables to meat and fish. Ancient Romans preserved fruit in honey. Salt has been used for centuries to cure meat and fish.

These methods of saving food for later use were simple and practical. But as the technology became more ingenious with time and the profit margin more revered, the processes became hazardous to our health. Salt, herbs, and spices were often used to disguise the odor and taste of rotting meat. Early experiments with metal cans resulted in many being poisoned by the lead used in the container. The use of boric acid as a preservative in the late 1800s was discovered to be toxic and removed. Incredibly, it was reinstated during the Second World War and was only finally banned in the 1950s. Boric acid has been associated with reproductive disorders in animal studies and is a suspected contributor to malformation of the foetus. The use of complex preservatives in our food is only half the additive story. The other half concerns flavor.

So, what do the people who make our food additives feel about them? Here is a statement about additives from the International Food Additives Council:

> The pursuit of happiness through the enjoyment of food is a centuries-old human endeavor. Taste, texture, freshness, and eye appeal are major contributors to such enjoyment, made possible in our modern lifestyle through the use of highly specialized ingredients known as food additives. Food additives afford us the convenience and enjoyment of a wide variety of appetizing, nutritious, fresh, and palatable foods. Their quantities in food are small, yet their impact is great. Without additives, we would be unfortunately lacking in the abundant and varied foods that we enjoy today.

The contention that additives ensure nutritious or fresh foods are particularly misleading. Why would you need preservatives if the food was fresh? The issue of appetizing and palatable additives only flies as long as you don't ask what it takes to make those foods taste and look the way they do. The additive business is all about deceit. The issue at hand is how do you make foods look, taste, and smell in a way that disguises their true condition. Let's peruse the International Food Additives Council for some more information. This quote is from one of their online information sheets:

> With well over 2,300 [this figure is estimated as between 3,000 and 5,000 by outside sources] food additives currently approved for use, it would be staggering to list the components of each of these substances. However, every additive—like every food we consume—no matter what its source or intended purpose, is composed of chemicals. Everything, including the clothes we wear, the cars we drive, the foods we eat, even our own bodies, is made up of chemicals.
>
> There is much discussion regarding "natural" and "synthetic" chemicals. Many of those synthesized in the laboratory are also found naturally occurring in foods. Chemicals are chemicals; **the distinction between a "natural" and "synthetic" chemical is itself artificial.** [The emphasis is mine.]

That's right, everything is made of chemicals, and it is too difficult to list all the ingredients—it's too complicated. They are right. It is true that everything is made of chemicals, but most people can understand the difference between a cabbage and a Volkswagen.

This old food additive cliché presents one of the primary disconnects in nutritional science—that food is simply a chemical delivery system, and that its effect on health is a result of understanding specific micronutrients. This narrow view has led us into decades of confusion and needless harm. It is also easily manipulated to prove almost any dietary theory. Of course, the food industry cherry-picks the science most likely to support consumption of the latest product.

A few years back, I was interviewed on a television show along with the late Dr Fredrick Stare, head of the Harvard University Department of Nutrition. He was a vocal critic of any dietary idea that was not generated by academics or industry, and he was a champion of the nutritional superiority and safety of the American food industry. What stands out in my mind was his becoming very agitated when I brought up the issue of organic agriculture. Apparently, he was not a big fan of nature. Here is a quote from an article he authored in *Life* magazine.

As a physician and as a student of nutrition for the last thirty years, I am convinced the food additives **are far safer in actual use than the basic natural foods themselves** [emphasis mine], because of improper food preparation, poor food habits, and overeating. The very few instances of harm from excessive or careless use of additives, or from their unanticipated effects, are overwhelmed by their many beneficial effects.

From the 1940s to the 1980s, Dr. Stare was a major voice on the topic of nutrition. He consistently defended the food industry and the American diet. While at Harvard, he defined the concept of the four major food groups: fruits and vegetables, grain products, milk products, and high-quality protein (meat). He was regarded as the voice of American nutritional science, and his basic message was that the food being manufactured by the modern food industry had the best nutritional value in human history. It was not until 1973 that Dr. Stare was exposed as a lobbyist for food, chemical, and pharmaceutical companies, some of whom had sponsored his work at Harvard.

THE AGE OF FAKE FLAVORS

The 1950s saw the emergence of the food "flavorist." The job of the flavor chemist was to duplicate the taste and fragrance of a natural food without the inconvenient need for the food itself. Making fruit drinks without fruit, bacon-flavored chips without any bacon, or a strawberry ice cream dessert that had never come within a mile of either a strawberry or cream was the challenge they happily accepted. It was a chemical game played with no attention to the health implications or transparency. The increased use of chemical flavors, dyes, and preservatives meant our foods were being adulterated at a level never before seen.

This was not a new issue. One early campaigner for food reform was the German chemist, Frederick Accum. In the early 1800s, he wrote a treatise on food adulteration that was a bestseller in England, Germany, and America. He regarded the counterfeiting and adulteration of food as a criminal offense. He wrote, *"The man who robs a fellow on the highway is sentenced to death, but he who distributes a slow poison to the whole community escapes unpunished.*" He also observed that the poisoning of the community generated huge wealth.

Accum discovered that there were dangerous and often fatal levels of many toxins in the food and drink of Londoners. Substances, such as red lead, mercury, copper, tin, sulfuric acid, chalk, wood chips, and even arsenic, were being used in everything from candy to cheese and bread to wine to color products, and also to disguise inferior food and drink.

If we fast-forward to 2014, we have a different list. The list below was compiled as part of the Master of Public Health Program at George Washington University. It is much longer than Accum's (this is called progress) and even more troubling. The Federal Food and Drug Agency (FDA) in America lists over three thousand chemical additives that are legal for commercial use. All are deemed safe by the people who make them and who also happen to be responsible for testing them.

Food Additives to Avoid

The George Washington University report says, "While FDA generally recognizes most additives on this list as 'safe,' there are growing concerns about the safety of many common food additives, if consumed in large quantities." This is the problem. Most of the chemicals used by industry to preserve food past the time it would decay or coverup the taste of a product that has the goodness processed out of it are toxic; we look the other way. We assume that the producer would never poison us. We are wrong. The list of "accepted" additions to our food are frightening.

- **Aluminum.** A preservative in some packaged foods that can cause cancer.

- **Azodicarbonamide.** Used in bagels and buns. Can cause asthma.

- **BHA/BHT.** A fat preservative, used in foods to extend shelf life. Linked to cancerous tumor growth.

- **Brominated vegetable oil.** Keeps flavor oils in soft drinks suspended. Bromate is a poison and can cause organ damage and birth defects. Not required to be listed on food labels.

- **Butane.** Put in chicken nuggets to keep them tasting fresh. A known carcinogen.

- **Carnauba wax.** Used in chewing gums and to glaze certain foods. Can cause cancer and tumors.

- **Carrageenan.** Stabilizer and thickening agent used in many prepared foods. Can cause ulcers and cancer.

- **Chlorine dioxide.** Used in bleaching flour. Can cause tumors and hyperactivity in children.

- **Disodium guanylate.** Used in snack foods, and it contains MSG.

- **Disodium inosinate.** In snack foods. Contains MSG.

- **Enriched flour.** Used in many snack foods. A refined starch that is made from toxic ingredients.

- **Magnesium sulphate.** Used in tofu, and it can cause cancer in laboratory animals.

- **Monosodium glutamate (MSG).** Flavor enhancer that can cause headaches. Linked in animal studies to nerve damage, heart problems, and seizures.

- **Olestra.** Fatlike substance that is unabsorbed by the body. Used in place of natural fats in some snack foods. Can cause digestive problems and is also not healthy for the heart.

- **Paraben.** Used to stop mold and yeast from forming in foods. Can disrupt hormones in the body, and it could be linked to breast cancer.

- **Polysorbate 60.** A thickener that is used in baked goods. Can cause cancer in laboratory animals.

- **Potassium bromated.** Added to breads to increase volume. Linked to cancer in humans.

- **Propyl gallate.** Added to fat-containing products. Linked to cancer in humans.

- **Propylene glycol.** Better known as antifreeze. Thickens dairy products and salad dressing. Deemed "generally" safe by the FDA.

- **Recombinant bovine growth hormone (rBGH).** Genetically engineered version of natural growth hormone in cows. Boosts milk production in cows. Contains high levels of IGF-1, which is thought to cause various types of cancer.

- **Refined vegetable oil.** Includes soybean oil, corn oil, safflower oil, canola oil, and peanut oil. High in omega-6 fats, which are thought to cause heart disease and cancer.

- **Sodium benzoate.** Used as a preservative in salad dressings and carbonated beverages. A known carcinogen and may cause damage to our DNA.

- **Sodium carboxymethyl cellulose.** Used as a thickener in salad dressings. Could cause cancer in high quantities.

- **Sodium nitrate.** Added to processed meats to stop bacterial growth. Linked to cancer in humans. (The worst offender.)

- **Sulfites.** Used to keep prepared foods fresh. Can cause breathing difficulties in those sensitive to the ingredient.

We should not wonder that each year more people say they are allergic to the foods they eat. All these chemicals are in the food that most people eat daily—in ever growing combinations that are completely untested except by the people who manufacture and use them.

Artificial Sweeteners to Avoid

Artificial sweeteners are regulated by the FDA, just as food additives are, but this does not apply to products "generally" recognized as safe. These additives are especially malicious since they fool the consumer into feeling they are avoiding the sugar they have been told is unhealthy. By replacing natural sugars with concentrated chemicals, the food companies can appeal to our natural desire for the sweet taste. In all cases the chemical does more damage to the body than the sugar would. It is all about profit not health.

- **Acesulfame potassium.** Used with other artificial sweeteners in diet sodas and ice cream. Linked to lung and breast tumors in rats.

- **Agave nectar.** Sweetener derived from a cactus. Contains high levels of fructose, which causes insulin resistance, liver disease, and inflammation of body tissues.

- **Aspartame.** An excitotoxin and thought to be a carcinogen. Can cause dizziness, headaches, blurred vision, and stomach problems.

- **Bleached starch.** Can be used in many dairy products. Thought to be related to asthma and skin irritations.

- **High-fructose corn syrup.** Sweetener made from corn starch. Made from genetically modified corn. Causes obesity, diabetes, heart problems, arthritis, and insulin resistance.

- **Saccharin.** Carcinogen found to cause bladder cancer in rats. (The worst offender.)

- **Sucralose.** "Splenda." Can cause swelling of liver and kidneys and a shrinkage of the thymus gland.

- **Tert-butylhydroquinone.** Used to preserve fish products. Could cause stomach tumors at high doses.

One of the most effective profit tools of the food industry is manufacturing foods to make a niche that is considered healthy. Producing Diet Drinks, Diet Dessert items, and Specialist Diabetic food items are a cynical strategy by the food industry to spread confusion and take advantage of the naive consumer.

Artificial Food Colorings to Avoid

Most modern food dyes are derived from petroleum. Again the purpose of the exercise is to fool the consumer. Would you eat grey salmon or grey peas? Would you eat canned vegetables with dull colors? No. What we see plays a big part in our response to food we are programmed to be suspicious of, foods that have the wrong color. Food manufacturers know this, and they simply test the colors that we like the best and paint the food accordingly.

- **Annatto.** Food coloring that can cause hyperactivity in children and asthma.

- **Bixin.** Food coloring that can cause hyperactivity in children and asthma.

- **Blue 1.** Used in bakery products, candies, and soft drinks. Can damage chromosomes and lead to cancer.

- **Blue 2.** Used in candies, beverages, and pet food. Can cause brain tumors.

- **Brown HT.** Used in many packaged foods. Can cause hyperactivity in children, asthma, and cancer.

- **Caramel coloring.** In soft drinks, sauces, pastries, and breads. When made with ammonia, it can cause cancer in mice. Food companies not required to disclose if this ingredient is made with ammonia.

- **Citrus red 1.** Sprayed on oranges to make them look ripe. Can damage chromosomes and lead to cancer.

- **Citrus red 2.** Used to color oranges. Can cause cancer if you eat the peel.

- **Green 3.** Used in candies and beverages. May cause bladder tumors.

- **Norbixin.** Food coloring that can cause hyperactivity in children and asthma.

- **Orange B.** A food dye that is used in hot dog and sausage casings. High doses are bad for the liver and bile duct.

- **Red 2.** A food coloring that may cause both asthma and cancer.

- **Red 3.** A carcinogen. Added to cherry pie filling, ice cream, and baked goods. May cause nerve damage and thyroid cancer.

- **Red 40.** Found in many foods to alter color. A carcinogen that is linked to cancer in some studies. Also can cause hyperactivity in children. Banned in some European countries. (The worst offender.)

- **Yellow 5.** Used in desserts, candies, and baked goods. Thought to cause kidney tumors, according to some studies.

- **Yellow 6.** A carcinogen used in sausages, beverages, and baked goods. Thought to cause kidney tumors, according to some studies.

You may have noticed how many of the known harmful effects of all the chemical preservatives, coloring agents, and general additives affect children the most. We are exposing our children to constant doses of unintended toxins on a daily basis. We should be worried about the accumulation of all these chemical challenges on the young. This is especially important since we have no idea what the accumulation of these chemicals is—no one has done studies.

BETTER LIVING THROUGH CHEMISTRY

As you can see, food scientists have been very busy providing us with convenience. Most of the additives in our food are only deemed safe at an imagined level of consumption; they are toxic at higher levels. The thinking is that "just a little bit of poison won't hurt you." The second issue we need to consider is that the ingredients in this chemical cocktail are all tested individually and not as they are used, in combination with other additives. Consider this: a Subway roasted chicken sandwich with cheese, mustard, and pickles on nine-grain bread will have at least 130 ingredients—including 30 chemical additives.

These chemicals are nutritionally useless. The human body has never encountered them over millions of years of evolution, yet we can easily consume up to a hundred of them a day. Americans spend about 90 percent of their food budget on processed foods. This equates to eating six to nine pounds of chemical additives a year.

Imagine your doctor offering you a pill containing a hundred ingredients and telling you that if you take one a day, your food will be tasty, but he has no idea of the physical damage that may occur.

To reiterate, since these chemicals are tested independently, we have no idea what happens when they are combined—and no one seems to be curious. One 2006 report published in *Toxicology Science* concluded that some common additives appeared to have neurotoxic effects when combined: *"Although the use of single food additives at their regulated concentrations is believed to be relatively safe in terms of neuronal development, their combined effects remain unclear."* Is this meant to reassure us? What does "relatively safe" mean? Is the increased prevalence of neurological disorders related to chemicals in the food? I don't know, you don't know, the food scientists don't know, and the manufacturers don't care.

The federal agency charged with protecting the public, the FDA, has no idea how many additives are being used. The testing of food additives is voluntary and self-regulatory. Companies are not compelled to tell the FDA about new ingredients prior to using it in a product. Talk about asking the fox to guard the henhouse! We have no idea how many additives are in actual use, but we know for sure that the list is littered with toxins and carcinogens.

The classification "generally recognized as safe" (GRAS) is the stamp of approval from the FDA for the safety of food additives. It is the equivalent of saying, "We guess it's OK. They told us it was." The United States Government Accountability Office (GAO) published a report in 2010 that was critical of the FDA and accused it of not ensuring the safety of food additives. They were particularly critical of the lack of supervision of new nanotechnology in food processing. This new technology involves the manipulation of matter at the molecular level. It might be considered similar to the genetic modification of plants or animals. No one knows the effect of these substances being used in food and packaging. You can see that willful ignorance is the default setting when it comes to health concerns. The FDA is so far behind the pace of the research, it doesn't even have the ability to test.

THE YUM-YUM FACTOR

These thousands of new chemical ingredients, together with advances in processing technology, are not only there to disguise the food but also to play on our senses. Food scientists discovered how to create a diet that actually makes us want to eat more. Their additives can trigger complex chemical reactions in us when we eat, and that makes us want to eat more and more—not only until we are full, but until we are stuffed.

One of the keys to this response is found in our evolution. During our early evolution, we had times of migration, when certain nutrients were in short supply. Among these were fat, simple sugars, and salt. When we eat foods that contain high concentrations of these substances, we want to gorge, since our primitive brain thinks we may not get them again soon. If we combine them, we have an even greater urge to consume them. Welcome to the modern diet.

The food industry can layer its products with scientifically determined amounts of salt, fat, and sugar to produce what they call "super-palatable" foods. These foods are easy to identify; they include anything where you open the package for "just a couple" and end up eating the whole bag. In the brave new world of nanotechnology, this will be done cheaply and without the base product.

With more consumers reading labels, manufacturers have simply become shrewd in their use of language. This is called "clean labelling." A shopper might notice that rosemary extract is an ingredient in salami. It might even be identified as natural or organic. That sounds very reassuring. "Rosemary extract" sounds much more natural than butylhydroxyansisoe (BHA) or butylhydroxytoluene (BHT)—both common chemical antioxidants that are used to slow down rancidity.

The problem is that the rosemary is dried and then passed through a chemical process using ethanol, hexane, and acetone, which removes all the taste and smell but isolates the antioxidant factors in the herb. What is produced is not even "rosemary-lite," but it certainly looks good on the label.

The high levels of sodium, sugar, and/or fat in processed food reduce your ability to taste subtler flavors. This is most dramatic with sugar. A shocking number of foods have added sugar. It is often used to disguise the taste of the salt. Many soups, snacks, and sauces, in addition to most fast foods, have huge quantities of sugar added, along with a strange mix of artificial ingredients.

Let's take a simple lunch at McDonald's for example. The number of calories in a McDonald's Happy Meal, including fries and a chocolate shake, is 1,090. It has 1,080 mg of sodium and 39 g of fat. (These figures come directly from the McDonald's website.) Here's the problem: the suggested caloric consumption for a child between the ages of 9 to 13 is 1,600 to 2,000 for a girl and 1,800 to 2,200 for a boy. This higher figure is for a child that is "moderately active." If sedentary, the lower figure is the guide. So on their Happy Meal day, a sedentary child can only have 400 calories of food to eat between breakfast and dinner.

The reason I pick children for the estimates is that they are the specific targets of McDonald's advertising. McDonald's is the largest distributor of toys in the world; their giveaways are a reason American children rank them as one of their favorite places to eat. The food industry likes to hook its customer at a very young age. We may call the food junk, but it's OK for the kids.

The results of eating this kind of a diet, and the nutritional stress associated with it, were predicted by many. Obesity, cancer, heart disease, and many illnesses that, in the past, had actually been rather rare, now became more and more common, particularly among the very young. This wasn't only in America but globally—everywhere the American food industry expands its nutritional empire. This calorically dense, nutritionally poor diet leaves a path of disease wherever it is introduced. Over the past fifty years, there has been a slow but rising awareness of this problem.

CAN WE TRUST THE SCIENCE?

I recently googled several food-related topics. "How to eat healthy" had 628,000,000 entries; "nutrition" had 632,000,000 results; "diet" had 1,010,000,000; and "what to eat" turned up 1,980,000,000! That's quite a bit of material to get through. With all that opinion, intellect, statistical data, science, and philosophy, no wonder we seem to be baffled by this simple question: What is a healthy diet?

Advertising supplies most of our "information" about the benefits of various foods. Every health concern (either real or imagined) requires a new product. If I sell cookies and can market the same basic product in a low-fat version, a gluten-free version, a sugar-free version, a natural version, and a diet version, I am laughing all the way to the bank. If I can persuade a nutritionist to say that the children's version has all the requirements for a healthy child, and a doctor to testify that the low-fat version is great for people with heart disease, I can drive sales through the roof.

Those who are afraid of potential health risks from food respond well to fear and simple answers. For every study that shows that dairy foods may be harmful, there is an industry study that touts milk. Every exposure of corporate dishonesty in producing a toxic food product is matched by a miracle nutrient pushed out in health food stores.

The public enchantment with "nutritional science" has created a flood of research sponsored directly by food manufacturers. A study in 1996 found that up to 30 percent of all university faculty members accepted funding from industry. With food scientists and researchers competing for money, the industry has found a willing extension to their PR departments. A study published in *PLoS Medicine* analyzed 206 publications on the health effects of various beverages, including milk, soft drinks, and fruit juices. Twenty-four of these studies had been funded solely by the industry whose product was investigated, and fifty-two of the papers declared that they had had no industrial support. The other papers had mixed support or did not declare sponsorship.

When studies were sponsored by a manufacturer of the beverage, a favorable result was four to eight times higher than those without corporate sponsorship. Out of the thirty-five interventional studies, which included human trials, industry was the sole sponsor of sixteen, and none of these sixteen reported an unfavorable outcome. The food activist Marion Nestle has estimated that up to 90 percent of nutritional research that is industry-sponsored favors the products tested. A problem is that food companies have the budget to assure that all positive studies reach the public. "Increasingly, nutrition science really isn't science," said Gary Ruskin, co-director of the food-industry watchdog group US Right to Know. "It's public relations." But the general public trusts science, so they believe the "scientifically proven information" and don't know when there is a hidden agenda.

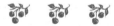

We do not need new products or even more studies to create a wholesome way of eating. What we need is a new way of looking at the whole issue of food and health. We need a user-friendly, common-sense approach to understanding food that is healthy and sustainable for society and the environment. To accomplish this requires us to question everything we have been told about nutrition and to review some very basic questions about the role of food in our life and in our culture.

Much of the modern food industry is based on creating an illusion. We are told to believe a food is healthy because it contains a magic ingredient or has had an offending one removed. We are easily lured by a colorful snack that is manufactured to resemble a childhood treat except it is only a chemical deception. If we are interested in our health and that of our family we have to learn to look behind the curtain and notice what the wizard has up his sleeve.

2

$\mathcal{S}$earching for the Silver Bullet

Science is the language of the modern age. It is only challenged by religion in terms of popular belief. Roughly four hundred years ago, science began its steady progress as a social force through insight and invention. The ruling belief in invisible forces driving religion was replaced by belief in the invisible force of numbers. The accusation of being "anti-science" is now a popular curse in the secular world and is used very flexibly to prove or disprove almost anything.

The attitude of scientific certainty in all matters is, unfortunately, wide of the mark. Science has produced astounding benefits but can be notoriously abused. The abuse usually comes from one of two sources. The first source of abuse is regarding the application of a discovery. It is possible to become excited and release something that is not tested or has negative long term effects.

The fact that inventions and insights are often best left till the implications of their use is fully understood is something that the rush to market often ignores. The second abuse has to do with who pays the bill. Science can be bought and sold. Quite often science that has been paid for is used to support a product or service that is harmful or fraudulent.

The interesting thing is that even when the valid (double blind, repeated, consistent peer reviewed) studies go counter to the status quo they are easily buried. Nutritional research often falls into this category. There is overwhelming proof showing that heart disease can be managed and even reversed through simple changes in lifestyle, and yet people are willing to take dangerous drugs to offset the symptoms. The

27

rate of diabetes in teens skyrockets; we know the cause, yet the problem "needs more study."

We suffer from a naive belief that science will come up with a pill or a miracle cure for all our ills but are reluctant to pay attention to what is already there. We have given away our ability to act before given expert permission.

If there is a thread of science that shows the safety of a medicine, the benefits of a food additive, or the stability of a melting ice-cap, we turn to a man or woman of science. If they say it's OK, we are on board. If the folks in the lab coats are in conflict, then it is too difficult for us to have an opinion or we can simply pick the belief we like best and stick with it.

ASKING THE WRONG QUESTION

The study of nutrition in ancient times was focused on the medicinal effects of foods. The kitchen was where nutritional science was born in making healing soups, stews, and teas. It was only in the nineteenth century that we started dissecting the food and looking for its hidden secrets. That approach helped solve many health problems. The links between diet and illnesses, such as scurvy, beriberi, anemia, and rickets, helped save lives and reduce misery. The great breakthroughs were about deficiencies.

The drive to discover "what's missing" continues to be an institutional prejudice in nutritional science. Nutrition researchers are always excited by the super-nutrient hiding in an obscure tropical fruit, or the single evil chemical lurking in a common vegetable. We are searching for outlaws and miracles.

Do We Need to Consume All the Antioxidants Flooding the Market?

Think of the recent popularity of antioxidants and their relationship to free radicals. The term "free radical" is appealing. It conjures the image of tiny bomb-wielding anarchists sneaking around our body. The war against free radicals prompted a mad rush to consume "antioxidants," who wore the white hats in this little drama. Of course, antioxidants are important. They balance off oxidative stress that can be produced by, for example, smoking, poor diet, environmental pollution, and exercise. Antioxidants prevent and repair the possible cell damage from free radical build-up.

Products with enough antioxidants to purge a herd of elephants flooded the market. Huge sales and increased price points followed. In reality, all that was required was for people to eat more colored fruits and vegetables. There are at least four thousand compounds that act as antioxidants in common fruits and vegetables. The daily requirement can be reached by eating a few vegetables with strong colors, such as carrots, broccoli, spinach, or berries.

The problem is that most nutritionally caused diseases in industrial societies are not caused by deficiencies at all. Excess is the issue. The overconsumption of a variety of foods eaten together causes our nutritionally dangerous diet. It is a perfect storm of chemicals, processed sugars, and animal fats and protein.

That doesn't stop nutritionists looking for the silver bullet. Every year, new and magical nutrients are discovered that will cure all ills. It might be an antioxidant, a specific protein, a fat, or a new vitamin—the information is always leveraged into the need for a new product, a dietary program, or to push a new best-selling book. This follows the same template used by the pharmaceutical industry: label a new disease and create a drug to treat it. This search for the miracle nutrient produces absurd arguments regarding the value of micronutrients that overshadow any serious discussion of healthy diets.

Are the Foods in the "Basic Four" Food Groups of Equal Value?

The standard American diet (SAD) serves as the model for the world food industry and is the best example of nutrition gone wrong. From 1956 through the 1990s, the most popular expression of nutritional needs was the "basic four" food groups. This template was built on the premise that meat, dairy, grain products, and vegetables were all of equal value and essential for good health. In other words, it was simply a rationalization of what was already being eaten. Those food groups erased all sense of food quality.

Meat was essential for "first-class" protein to build the body. Dairy was needed to provide calcium for bone growth, as well as more protein and some vitamins. Breads and breakfast cereals would provide energy and fiber, and vegetables would supply the vitamins.

The absurdity of this approach was demonstrated in the early 1980s when the Department of Agriculture (USDA) Food and Nutrition Service, under Ronald Reagan, produced school lunch guidelines to fit the regulations. Students could have a half pint of milk (dairy requirement) and a small hamburger patty (meat requirement) on a bun (grain requirement) with relish (vegetable requirement). The pickle relish as the vegetable only really raised a storm when it was suggested that it could be replaced with ketchup. "Ketchup—a vegetable? Crazy!" But the idea fit the understanding of nutritional standards. Everyone knows that fruits and vegetables are healthy and should go somewhere in the diet; grandmothers all over the world tell children to make sure to eat their vegetables. Although an important side dish, it was the other three groups that were essential.

The application of those nutritional guidelines regarding the use of cereal grains provides an insight into the absurdity of this method of understanding food. Grain was and still is included in the plates, pyramids, and pie charts that make up nutritional graphics. They are usually illustrated by a loaf of bread, a bowl of breakfast cereal, maybe a bowl of white rice or pasta, and—when "carbohydrate" is used instead of grain—a potato makes an appearance.

MORE THAN A GRAIN OF TRUTH

No distinction is made between an actual whole grain and a supposedly whole-grain product. This is the USDA definition of whole-grain foods according to the Whole Grains Council.

Foods must meet one of three requirements:

- Contain at least 8 g of whole grain content per serving, or

- Qualify for FDA whole grain health claim (51 percent whole grain by weight), or

- Have a whole grain as the first ingredient, or the first grain ingredient by weight for non-mixed dishes (for example, breads, cereals) or as the first grain ingredient for mixed dishes (such as, pizza, corn dogs)

- In essence, at least 50 percent of the grain must be whole grain.

So it is not the case that whole grain means "whole grain." If my math is right, 50 percent of the grain being "whole grain" gives you "half grain." This is an advertising con, not a nutritional requirement. Food manufacturers do not want you to know too much about what is in your food; they simply want you to feel good about eating it.

Grain that has been ground, pressed, rolled, or popped is as different from actual whole grain as night is from day. The application of heat and the cracking of the outer layers of the dry grain bring about nutritional degradation almost instantly. The oils in the grain begin to go rancid, and the oxidation exacerbates the breakdown of vitamins and protein. This process happens over a period of weeks. This is very relevant since most Americans and Europeans eat bread and flour products made with refined product. And we eat a lot of it: the average American eats 53 lb. of bread a year. (That doesn't include cakes, pizzas, cookies, and pastas.)

USDA figures for the year 2000 demonstrate part of the problem. Total grain consumption rose from 155 lb. a year in the 1950s to just under 200 lb. in 2000. That should be a happy fact except that only 7 percent of the population were eating whole grain as opposed to processed grain.

Grain has gained a bad reputation in the past few years because of how it is processed and mixed with other ingredients. Most research has shown that people who eat a diet with whole grains are healthier than those who don't. In fact, if you had to choose only one food to live on for the rest of your life, you couldn't do better than whole cereal grains. It is not that they are a "superfood," but they cover many of the basic human nutritional needs. They aren't sexy, but they are reliable.

A recent study from a Harvard Medical School team tracked over 367,000 healthy people who were taking part in the NIH-AARP Diet and Health Study over a period of fourteen years. People with preexisting conditions were excluded. Participants were quizzed about their diets, exercise habits, and other lifestyle factors; they were also monitored for health conditions and mortality.

Those people who ate more whole grains had a 17 percent reduced risk of death, compared to those who ate much less. When it came to the cereal fiber itself, people who ate the most had a 19 percent reduced risk of death from any cause, compared to those who ate the least. People who ate the most cereal fiber had 15 percent and 34 percent reduced risk of death from cancer and diabetes respectively. This is a consistent result from studies throughout the past decades and from around the world. But what about the trend to demonize gluten?

Gluten Intolerance

The sudden appearance of celiac disease and gluten intolerance as health concerns over the past decade requires a few remarks. Gluten is a protein found in a number of cereal grains. The common offenders are wheat, rye, barley, spelt, triticale, and products derived from them. The prevalence of Celiac Disease in the United States and most European countries has been identified as 0.71 percent of the population. The number of people thought to have a gluten intolerance (but not CD) is a similar number. Most of those people have not been formally diagnosed. Most people who were following a gluten-free diet did not have Celiac Disease.

There is no question that some people have CD (which can be confirmed by taking an antibody test), gluten intolerance, or other poor reactions to the above mentioned grains. The symptoms of bloating, diarrhea or chronic constipation, fatigue, or irritability are certainly worrying; and serious damage to the intestinal wall can occur with CD. If these people do not have CD or GI why do they present the symptoms when flour is consumed?

If we look at the fact that only 7 percent of the American population were eating "whole" as opposed to "refined" grain, we get an important insight. Most of the refined products are manufactured along with sugars, yeast, oils, trans fats, and a very wide range of other additives. These products produce excessive digestive stress, which contributes to immune dysfunction. The actual consumption of whole grains or unadulterated grain products is not part of the assessment.

My experience in working with hundreds of clients who have been told that they are gluten-sensitive or intolerant is that if they change to a less stressful diet that eliminates the refined and adulterated products, most can add whole grain into their diet with no problems.

Complex Carbohydrates

Complex carbohydrates provide energy and are rich in proteins, healthy fats, minerals, vitamins, enzymes, and fiber. Complex carbohydrates are made into glucose (blood sugar) in the intestines. Glucose is what the body runs on. When the complex carbohydrates found in grains and vegetables are eaten, the sugars are digested and absorbed slowly into the body. They can be used when needed and stored easily. They also contain all the other nutrients (minerals, vitamins, and fiber) essential for the sugars to be utilized.

Many people imagine that eating grain will make them gain weight, but observing grain-eating cultures show that is not the case. It is the kind of carbohydrate we eat that makes the difference. When sugars are refined and isolated, we have problems. Sharp rises in blood sugar are associated with refined sugars. Excessive sugar in the diet, particularly of the refined varieties, means that the glucose must be stored in the form of glycogen. It is dishonest to demonize all sugars "carbs" and then disregard the actual need for carbohydrates in their natural form.

The fact that our body runs on glucose (a sugar) brings up the next aspect (and one of the most perplexing) of the SAD diet: sugar. Sugar is the single dietary component that people recognize as harmful, and yet it is one of the most cherished. When talk turns to dessert, the conversation is passionate. It is always interesting to see the response when someone is asked to remove simple sugars from their personal menu. It is as if an old friend has passed away or happiness will disappear. We are well and truly hooked; sugar is the most common drug of choice.

FOOD FIGHTS—SUGAR CONSUMPTION

Once again, confusion is the friend of the food business. One of the prime composers of this confusion was our old friend Fredrick Stare who founded the Department of Nutrition at Harvard School of Public Health. The Department of Nutrition at Harvard was pulling in large sums of money from the sugar industry. From 1953 to 1956, the Sugar

Research Foundation, established by the sugar refiners, cited thirty papers from Harvard funded by them. In 1960, the university began work on a $5 million building funded by General Foods, among other members of Big Food. Regular donors to Stare's empire were Coca-Cola, Kellogg, Gerber, and Oscar Mayer. Harvard was becoming the voice of the American food industry.

Still, a growing number of people criticized the use of sugar. The sugar industry needed Stare and his department to reassure the public, via governmental agencies, to continue its sugar consumption. The Food and Nutrition Advisory Council compiled "Sugar in the Diet of Man," an eighty-eight-page white paper edited by Stare was published in 1975. The task was to "organize existing scientific facts concerning sugar." It was a compilation of historical evidence and arguments that sugar companies could use to counter the claims of British professor John Yudkin, who had emerged as a dangerous foe of the industry. Stare's study was funded by the industry. If this reminds you of all the misinformation from "reliable scientific sources" that surrounded the efforts of the tobacco industry to suppress negative research, you wouldn't be far off. Some of the same players were involved in that particular scam.

Much of the panic was a response to the research of Yudkin and his Department of Nutrition at the University of London. Yudkin was the preeminent nutritionist of his generation in the UK. He established the first ever degree course in nutrition in Europe. In 1972, Yudkin published *Pure, White, and Deadly*—a reflection on his decades of research on the dangers of sugar. The book was a best seller in the UK, and it was published in America as *Sweet and Dangerous* (the word "deadly" was a step too far for the American publishers). It was widely translated and circulated. It established Yudkin as the "enemy" of the sugar industry.

Yudkin's premise was that sugar was implicated in a wide range of illnesses, including diabetes and coronary thrombosis. He linked these diseases to the sharp rise in insulin that accompanied sugar consumption. He correctly identified it as a food additive, not a natural ingredient. Referring to the lack of serious research on the effects of sugar, he said, *"If only a small fraction of what we know about the effects of sugar were to be revealed in relation to any other material used as a food additive, it would be banned."*

Following the publication of his book, Yudkin's professional life became miserable. Invitations to conferences on nutrition (increasingly sponsored by the food industry) were cancelled, and many articles in the popular press attacked his "science fiction" approach to nutrition. The food industry has consistently used this same strategy of personal attacks on its critics.

The second worrying voice for the sugar industry was a journalist named William Dufty. I knew Dufty, a tireless advocate for a healthy diet and an insightful social critic. He was instrumental in introducing macrobiotics to American audiences with *You Are All Sanpaku*, his translation of the writing of George Oshawa. *Sugar Blues* is a classic in the alternative approach to nutrition and has sold over 1.5 million copies.

In many ways, Dufty's book had more impact than Yudkin's in America. Dufty was a journalist who was no stranger to investigative reporting; he knew a crooked deal when he saw it. He had no academic credentials to protect. He was after the truth. In keeping with the macrobiotic philosophy, he addressed the impact of sugar politically and socially, as well as its impact on health. He discussed it as a drug, not a food. These men, Yudkin and Dufty, were important pioneers in the movement toward a healthy diet. They raised an alarm about a toxic product that had become a favorite ingredient in the manufacturing of processed food.

The increased use of sugar and chemical food additives are two of the most striking aspects of the modern diet. According to the United States Department of Agriculture (USDA), the average American eats between 150 lb. And 170 lb. of refined sugar each year. That is compared to about the 4 lb. consumed one hundred years ago. Remember: that's an average. Someone out there is eating over 200 lb. or more and suffering the effects.

A variety of studies have shown that consuming only 75 g to 100 g of simple sugar (about the amount found in two and a half cans of soda) can suppress the body's immune responses considerably. The sugars create a 40 percent to 50 percent drop in the ability of white blood cells to kill bacteria and germs within the body. This immune-suppressing effect of sugar takes place within thirty minutes and may last for hours.

I have pointed to the dangers of sugar and additives. Let's look at two more foods that have been darlings of conventional nutrition since its inception: meat and dairy. Meat and dairy have been the foundation blocks of American food. They are claimed to make us strong, muscular, alert, and maybe even manly.

MAN THE HUNTER—MEAT CONSUMPTION

It is easy to see that the extent of meat consumption was originally a reflection of weather, soil, and environmental conditions when viewed through the lens of history. If there were plentiful fruits, nuts, seeds, berries, edible leaves, and tubers, we were fairly content. If the growth was sparse and the climate cold, and the growing season short, the consumption of the fats in meat—and later in dairy foods—would naturally increase. The vision we have of the meat-eating tradition is hazy. But we do know that, today, America is the all-time champion of meat consumption.

As early as 1861, the novelist Anthony Trollope reported that Americans ate twice the amount of beef as the English. When Charles Dickens visited, he reported, "No breakfast was breakfast without a T-bone steak." Once the early settlers established a foothold in America, they were faced with a continent bursting with life. Innumerable wild birds and mammals crowded the plains and forests. Grazing lands stretched as far as the eye could see. Abundant meat, historically the privilege of the very wealthy was now available to most families. This did not last, but the idea of eating meat daily still reverberates in the American psyche and is still associated with success. The wealthy grill a steak, the poor have hamburger.

Nutritional science supported the importance of meat by claiming it as a "first-class protein"—food for the muscles. Vegetables, of course, were needed but meat was the "real deal." We now comprehend the link between animal products and the increases in heart disease, stroke, cancers, and even diabetes. What urges us to eat meat as even a small part of a healthy diet? Many believe that eating meat is hardwired into our biology, but it would be more accurate to say it has been psychology and imagination that play the important roles. Several images may spring to mind:

- The brave hunter returns to the cave with an antelope strapped on his back, which he offers to his family as they cower in the shadows of their cave.

- The independent cowboy hunkers down beside the campfire for a big plate of fried meat and cornbread.

- The wealthy landowner sits down to the groaning table filled with roasted birds, fishes, and legs of lamb.

- Dad fires up the grill and throws on the steaks. The flags are flying.

Powerful images that operate below the surface of consciousness often define what we do. Man the hunter, rugged individualism, dominion over the earth, power over ignorant animals, wealth, and shared experience—these all form, in part, our attitudes to food. What arguments could be used to justify this habit that is creating illness, brutality, and ecological ruin? The answer is a heady mix of bad science, cultural myopia, and a fear of change.

One of the most interesting arguments supporting the eating of meat is that we are omnivorous. I would never argue with that. Early humans ate a varied diet that probably included insects, small game, fruits, and plants. The road from our ancient origins has many twists and turns. What serves survival along the way may not be essential in our present location. There are many things that I can do, that I choose not to do now. There are many things I have done that I don't wish to do again. Respecting ancestors doesn't require repeating their mistakes. Isn't that how we learn?

Some commentators on the history of human diets claim we are actually carnivores. A carnivore is an animal that has a diet mainly or exclusively of animal meat. This meat can be obtained through either hunting and killing or scavenging the leftovers from what other animals kill. The academic arguments continue regarding the dietary details of our evolution, but certain compelling facts emerge that challenge our cultural mythologies.

Are We True Carnivores?

The most accurate indications of early diet are to be found in our own mouth and intestinal tract. This is where the history of any animal's dietary past is reflected most dramatically. Indications of the earliest human remains show that man was never a true carnivore. In fact, meat (other than insects) was probably a rather small part of dietary consumption. The proofs of this lie in both human structure and function.

Starting with the most obvious, our so-called canine teeth don't qualify us as carnivores. They are placed back toward the outer corners of the mouth. They are not long enough, large enough, or strong enough to grip, hold, and tear flesh. They most certainly are teeth designed for holding food. There is no evidence in the fossil record that we have ever had the sharp, developed teeth to tear meat, or the jaw joints to hold the kill with any effectiveness—alone the claws that are essential tools for the capture of prey. Most people can barely open plastic packets with their fingernails, let alone puncture the hide of a struggling animal.

The issue of cheeks often brings a laugh when I am teaching. I guess there is something intrinsically amusing about cheeks. Carnivores don't have them. They don't need them. You don't keep meat in your mouth; you only have cheeks when you keep food in your mouth to mix with saliva and to masticate. Humans have digestive enzymes in our mouth to digest complex carbohydrates (not needed for carnivores). We do not develop this capacity unless it is essential to our existence. The same indications exist in the human intestinal tract.

Carnivores have very short intestines with fairly smooth walls. Meat fiber is not beneficial to intestinal health in any animal, so when the surface nutrients are released from meat, the intestines need to be flushed. Herbivores and humans have a longer (two to three times as long), more complex digestive tract that holds vegetable fiber for significantly more time to achieve maximum efficiency and support the growth of beneficial microorganisms. All these features take us back over several hundred million years, to a period long before the development of tools or the common use of fire.

Our Ability to Adapt

One of our most precious gifts is our adaptability, so it is difficult to interpret the indications of our original diet. The first humans left their African home 1.8 to 1.3 million years ago. As we travelled, and as other waves of migration worked their way north, we were forced to adapt to new environments. As tribes moved into the colder and less fertile lands, they followed herds of animals and relied more on animal sources of food for survival. Tribes that remained in the cooler climates—high mountains where the soil was poor or in areas where edible foods were scarce—kept using animals as a food source. Many eventually domesticated animals and used them for milk products.

Adaptation is the force behind our physical evolution, but adaptation also happens on a cultural level. The cultural influence is usually expressed through innovation. Some innovation came through developing the use of fire, cooking, clothes, shelter, food fermentation and developing tools to hunt. These early innovations were well established as long as three hundred thousand years ago, during the Palaeolithic period. The skills and tools provided protection from attack or the vagaries of the climate and they fed us. We ate what was available, and it was certainly "local, seasonal, and mostly fresh."

People ate what was available. But the mythology of "man the hunter" is quite misleading. The archaeological records, as well as human physiology, tell a different story. With more recent discoveries using advanced technology, we now see that many (perhaps most) of our ancestors ate significant amounts of plant food. An international team of archaeologists from Haifa University, Bar-Ilan University, Hebrew University, and Harvard, discovered a site on the shores of the Sea of Galilee where primitive agriculture was being practiced 23,000 years ago. They were even grinding their own flour. This is about 13,000 years before agriculture was thought to be practiced.

Over the following centuries, our innovations had a tendency to focus on the tools of hunting, war, and the manufacture of garments and decorations. It is unclear how frequently we used fire for cooking, although it certainly happened. There is evidence of humans using fire that date back 1 million years and perhaps earlier. Fire was evidenced in cooking hearths and earth ovens from between 500,000 and 300,000 years ago. This evidence is spread through Europe and the Middle East. There are many scholars who go so far as to state that cooking was a prime influence in human physical and mental development. This theory notes that cooking food increases its caloric impact and releases excess energy which would be used in digestion.

The Agricultural Revolution

Human life was still governed by the seasons and the local ecosystem. All that started to change radically between 10,000 BC and 6,000 BC with the agricultural revolution. In areas as diverse as the Middle East, China, and the Americas, people started settling in one place and growing their own food. People needed foods that could feed the largest numbers from the least land. Grains, beans, and tubers became the focus of human food. They all required cooking. We cooked to soften the fibers and increase the availability of nutrients in them.

The rise of agriculture meant we needed to understand nature in a different way. We moved from reacting to nature into a particular partnership with it. Farmers selected specific strains of plants best suited for human consumption and started growing them. This involved creating an environment for their growth. Humans started to nourish the soil, irrigate the fields, save seeds, and select the heartiest plants. This was how our present-day grains, beans, vegetables, and animal breeds originated. We began to create a sustainable method of eating that allowed us to develop a culture quite different from our nomadic existence.

When I ask clients to describe their diet, the two most common answers are "I eat a really good diet" (everything is relative) and "I was raised on a traditional diet, I like my meat and potatoes." The former is usually the female answer, and the latter comes mostly from men. Tradition is used as a reason for a multitude of sins. If it was good enough for Grandpa, it's good enough for me. But is our nostalgia for tradition a reflection of reality or a fantasy? And what is the value of tradition per se?

When I started to eat a macrobiotic diet my grandfather told me that I was eating more like he did as a child. His family lived on porridge, bread, vegetables, beans, and small game, with very little red meat. He thought what I was doing was amusing, and he loved the food. Most people ate very little meat a hundred years ago. While Darwin was eating his steak, most people were eating more grains and vegetables. I have found this to be true in every country I have visited. If you ask the elders, their diet included less meat unless they were quite wealthy.

There has been a long association between wealth and meat eating. This is still true today; meat eating and the abundance of food are often associated with success. It has always been the rich who were overweight, but now the tables are turning. Using government subsidies, environmentally damaging practices, and complete disregard for the welfare of the animals has produced plentiful cheap meat and dairy. These are now the staples of the fast-food diet. These foods are calorie rich and nutrient deficient.

According to a survey of available research done by the Physicians Committee for Responsible Medicine, countries with a higher intake of fat—especially fat from animal products, such as meat and dairy products—have a higher incidence of breast cancer.

Foods high in animal fats are thought to disrupt the hormonal balance in women and increase estrogen production. You will find a listing of more studies in Chapter Thirteen. I love this quote from the January 2015 issue of *Discover* magazine (Science for the Curious):

> Humans are the only carnivores that face an increased risk of cancer as a result of eating red meat, but no one really knew why. . . . It's not all bad news. Researchers said that red meat is an important source of iron, proteins, and other vitamins; so moderate red meat consumption does yield nutritional benefits.

What a close call. Meat gives you cancer, but you will not suffer from anemia.

Scientific Findings

Recent studies have shown that cooked meat contains concentrations of heterocyclic amines (HCAs), a mutagenic compound. HCAs are produced when meat is cooked, and they are linked with the development of many cancers. These compounds are found in higher concentrations when meat is cooked at higher temperatures, such as when grilled or fried.

A Harvard Health Professionals cohort study on diet and prostate cancer risk reported on almost fifty-two thousand health professionals. The study was based on food frequency questionnaires in 1986. After three to four years of follow-ups, it was found that there was a significant risk of prostate cancer with those who ate the most red meat. It was the meat consumption that was the most significant association with advanced prostate cancer. This is only a sample of the many findings that indicate the relationship between prostate cancer and meat consumption.

No matter how dire the news is on meat, we continue consuming it. The popular fast-food hamburger can contain as little as 15 percent meat and includes bones, connective tissue, blood vessels, fat, water, nerves, cartilage, and plant-based fillers. No one wants to know what's in a hot dog. So-called traditions of meat-eating serve those who sell meat but are not a reflection of reality.

There is an irony in the clarion call for "survival of the fittest"—a term that Darwin borrowed from Herbert Spencer. The fitness referred to is the capacity to successfully reproduce, and yet it is those modern meat-eating cultures that are exhibiting a 50 percent reduction in sperm count over the past sixty years and reduced fertility in women.

The question still hangs in the air. Even if our ancestors ate meat as their primary food, why should that affect our diet today? An important aspect of eating is survival; our present consumption of meat is moving us away from survival and into sickness and, perhaps, extinction.

THE DAIRY DECEPTION

Milk products are almost sacrosanct in America and much of Europe. Everyone knows that milk helps children grow big and strong, and that if you don't drink milk you may develop problems with your bones. For many years, this was the message from nutritionists and the medical profession. It came as a big shock when the studies started flooding in that the opposite was true—particularly regarding osteoporosis.

If you are like me, you grew up being told that milk was an essential part of the human diet. We were taught that if you didn't drink milk, you would have "weak bones," because milk had lots of calcium. What if we ask the question "What *is* it?" rather than "What's *in* it?"

All female mammals produce milk, a nutrient-rich food produced specifically to help the young develop in a healthy manner. The milk not only contains the specific nutrients needed but also the immune factors essential for the young of the species to survive. This is true of the cow and the human mother, the mouse, and the kangaroo. The milk of each species is perfect for the new-born of that species and reflects specific requirements.

A human baby usually does not walk till about eleven to fourteen months after birth. Before that time, they are carried or crawling. It may be as long as sixteen months to two years before a child can run. The greatest development during this period is in the brain and nervous system.

The size of a human baby's brain doubles in the first year, and by age three, it has reached 80 percent of its adult volume. What is more important is that the number of synapses (the connecting fibers in the brain) develop faster than at any other time in our lives. We develop twice as many of these microscopic connections than we will retain. We are very busy during our first two years of life creating a brain that can manage a huge amount of information. We are getting ready to think, not to run. Human milk is especially suited to brain growth. Babies who are breastfed have been shown to have higher scores in neurodevelopment and cognition in later life.

When we look at the early life of the calf, we see a very different emphasis in growth. A calf stands and walks within ten minutes to an hour of birth. This is essential since a cow has evolved to move with the herd. It is part of its evolutionary life pattern. The calf needs long, strong bones. It doesn't really increase much brain size or complexity during its infancy. The brain size of a human baby at birth is almost 70 percent of the adult size of the brain, but his body weight is only 5 percent of an adult's. During the first year of life, 15 percent brain growth occurs—thus the need for breastfeeding is to enhance brain growth. The huge concentration of calcium in cow's milk is often used as an advertising gimmick, but it only makes sense if the focus is on overall body size and not brain function.

Cow's milk is food to grow a healthy cow. I was raised on drinking milk daily. My mother was following the advice of every doctor and dietician of the times; the requirement (not option) of drinking milk was understood as scientific fact—it was not. But now the "facts" are being rewritten.

Scientific Findings

Dr. David Ludwig and Dr. Walter Willett from Harvard University published a study in the *Journal of the American Medical Association* refuting government proposals for dairy consumption. The Harvard scientists found no data to support the claim that the consumption of dairy leads to bigger bones, weight loss, or improved health. They also found some serious risks tied to dairy consumption, including weight gain, increased cancer risk, and incredibly, given that milk was supposed to strengthen our bones, increased fracture risk.

Clinical research shows that dairy products have little or no benefit for bones. A 2005 review published in *Pediatrics* showed that milk consumption does not improve bone integrity in children. The Harvard Nurses' Health Study, which followed more than seventy-two thousand women for eighteen years, showed no protective effect of increased milk consumption on fracture risk.

According to the Nurses' Health Study, the risk of fracture is *increased* by up to 50 percent with dairy consumption. Less dairy equals better bones. Countries with the lowest rates of dairy and calcium consumption, like those in Africa and Asia, have the lowest rates of osteoporosis. Those with high consumption have the highest rates of the disease.

Dr. Neal Barnard, nutrition researcher, stated, "What appears to be important in bone metabolism is not calcium intake, but calcium balance. The loss of bone integrity among many postmenopausal white women probably results from genetics and from diet and lifestyle factors. Research shows that calcium losses are increased by the use of animal protein, salt, caffeine, and tobacco, and by physical inactivity."

About 65 percent of the world's population is genetically unable to properly digest milk. This condition is called lactose intolerance. I have seen this referred to as a disorder. I see it as a gift.

Health Risks

The financial force of a food product overrides all health considerations. The *"Got Milk"* campaign aimed at children and the "milk mustache" campaign were aimed at "reinforcing the drink's nutritional value with young mothers and twentysomething buyers." The campaigns in America were done under government supervision to bolster the industry in a slumping milk market. Yet they knew that the claims about milk as a "health food" and building strong bones were completely contradicted by the science. The money wasn't only talking, it was shouting.

Eventually, in response to questions raised by the Physicians Committee for Responsible Medicine, a scientific review of the milk claims was released by the US Department of Agriculture. It offered support for critics who claimed that the dairy industry overstated milk's nutritional merits.

The USDA-appointed panel concluded that milk cannot be considered a "sports drink," does not specifically prevent osteoporosis, and—in its high-fat, whole-milk form—might play a role in heart disease and prostate cancer. Since the milk industry spent $190 million on the milk ads and the USDA report didn't even make the front page of the papers for one day, not much happened. The news about the dangers of dairy consumption has not offset industry-sponsored propaganda.

As stated (meekly) in the report, the relationship between dairy foods and osteoporosis is only one of the health dangers of milk products. Breast and prostate cancers have also been linked to consumption of dairy products, presumably related, at least in part, to increases in a compound called insulin-like growth factor (IGF-1). IGF-1 is found in cow's milk and has been shown to occur in increased levels in the blood of individuals consuming dairy products on a regular basis.

The dairy industry has one of the most impressive propaganda machines in the food industry. Americans and Western Europeans love milk and milk products. According to Food Democracy, the average American consumes 31 lb. of cheese, 600 lb. of non-cheese dairy products, and 181 lb. of beverage milk per year. This total of 812 lb. is a very substantial portion of the 1,996 lb. of food that the individual will eat in a year.

As usual, there is a search for the silver bullet. The path of that search is endless and circular. For every micronutrient or compound that is found to be harmful, another can be dredged up that has some benefit. Always in the background are the financial interests that create new products and mold the public desire for them.

THE BIG PICTURE

Fortunately, there is one field of nutritional research that has consistently cast a light on the problems with the modern diet; that's epidemiology. This is the study of large groups of people, their habits, and the outcomes. Researchers observe how people behave and then see if they can identify correlations between behavior and health. For over forty years, epidemiological studies have been sending up a warning signal about dairy products. Few have paid attention—not the medical practitioners.

Much of the focus in epidemiology has been on the prevalence of NCDs (noncommunicable diseases). These diseases cause 85 percent of American deaths. The world average is higher than that, and at current rates, by the year 2030, NCD's will cause 89 percent of all deaths in America.

The epidemiological information about foods that make us sick and those that are productive of health has not changed at all. So why is so little action taken? Major universities and medical schools are changing their tune at a rapid rate. The following is from a 2009 Harvard University newsletter.

> Traditionally, research into vegetarianism focused mainly on potential nutritional deficiencies, but in recent years, the pendulum has swung the other way. Nowadays, plant-based eating is recognized as not only nutritionally sufficient but also as a way to reduce the risk for many chronic illnesses. In July 2009, the American Dietetic Association weighed in with a position paper, concluding that "appropriately planned vegetarian diets, including total vegetarian or vegan diets, are healthful, nutritionally adequate, and may provide health benefits in the prevention and treatment of certain diseases."

We are getting important information about what causes the diseases that kill us, and yet we don't do anything about it. Even worse, governments actively support the very foods that are most damaging. Some of this support is in the publication of industry influenced "Dietary Goals" but more importantly, far from the public eye, is the direct financial support of subsidies.

Between 1995 and 2010 the American government spent $170 billion in agricultural subsidies to finance the production of food. The largest section of this expense was the "big seven." These crops and farm foods are: corn, soybeans, wheat, rice, sorghum, milk, and meat. Only a small portion of the crops listed are used as human food. Most of the subsidies are directly used for animal feed, processed into biofuels, cheap additives, such as corn sweeteners, industrial oils, and refined products.

In a 2011 report by the U.S. Public Interest Research Group the targeted expenditure on junk food additives from the above total was $18 billion. That money went to corn syrup, high fructose corn syrup, corn starch, and soy oils processed into hydrogenated vegetable oils. Tax money is being used to subsidise the very industries that are making us sick.

Our resistance to dietary reform is certainly not driven by logic or science. If our refusal to change were only damaging ourselves, if it really was an individual decision, I would say that it is each person's free choice. We can commit suicide with our fork if we want to. But the problem goes much deeper than that. In order for nutritional reform to take place, there has to be some radical change in the scientific community and the medical profession. Doctors are on the front line of our health-care systems and form a wall of opposition to any challenge to their monopoly on health information. It is a sad fact that the wall is manufactured from inexperience, professional myopia, and arrogance.

This resistance is especially tragic because it is directly related to the increased incidence of those diseases that are likely to cause our death. The frequency of heart disease, diabetes, and many cancers are on the rise. Modern health requires the most urgent reformation and the clock is ticking.

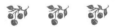

What becomes obvious is that the food we eat outstrips any other single lifestyle or environmental cause of disease. This terrible situation has been caused in great part by the search for "what's missing." That peculiar prejudice on the part of nutrition has driven research (often with a pre-determined goal) and practice for almost 100 years. It still is a major factor not only in conventional practice but also among so-called alternative practitioners. We want an easy answer, a magical supplement, a superfood. Once identified it will be marketed and last until the new one comes along. The coconut fades into the avocado and then moves into the turmeric. The answer may be much simpler than we imagine.

The most important development over the past twenty years has been the clear message regarding sugar, milk and meat. They are not only a poor choice for good nutrition but may well be the primary cause of many of our diseases. If a solid basis of prevention is followed we may avoid many of the degenerative processes that plague society. If that route is not taken then another set of barriers face us in the form of the medical orthodoxy. This should be where a new health oriented path is revealed to us. Unfortunately, as we will see, that is not always the case.

3

$\mathscr{B}$ad Medicine

onventional medicine has a sad and dysfunctional relationship with nutrition. Growing evidence on connections between diet and disease means doctors are asked questions they have evaded for decades. Many of my clients experiencing the benefits of a healthy plant-based diet ask, "Why didn't my doctor know about this?" There is not one answer to this question, there are many and all contribute to a worrying trend in health care.

I fully respect the good work that most doctors do. Modern medicine can do many wonderful things. But medicine is rarely criticized or assessed rigorously from the outside. I have witnessed medical bullying and it is not pretty. When a mother asked questions regarding a procedure on one of her children the doctor brushed the question aside. He said, "Are you a doctor? If not you should leave the medicine to me." We need to ask questions and get answers when our health or that of our family is on the line. There are mythologies surrounding medicine that are deeply embedded in our culture, and these profoundly affect our attitudes to health, including nutrition.

Since the 1950s, medical shows on television have been standard entertainment; at the last count, there have been ninety-three successful shows in America (thirty-two in the UK) with a medical format. From *Dr. Kildare* and *Ben Casey* in the 1960s to *ER* and *House* in the twenty-first century, television doctors have portrayed the power of medicine over suffering and death. But it is a mistake to believe that this power indicates that doctors understand health. They are sickness experts, not health experts.

HEALTH EXPERTS VS SICKNESS EXPERTS

The difference between health experts and sickness experts is important. The focus of all medical training is on treatment not prevention. Doctors are trained to diagnose and prescribe—that is the focus of all their learning. We want our doctors to know what to do in the case of serious illness, but we cannot afford the medical myopia that now exists. This is particularly true when most of the diseases that kill us can be prevented before they advance to the stage where treatment is required.

It is not a particular failing by individual doctors that is the issue. It is the institution of medicine that is at fault, as well as the public resistance to change. Medical research into the impact of nutrition in the creation of disease is overwhelming and so is growing evidence of the role of diet in reversing many health problems. In the face of this information, what is stopping doctors from telling their patients how to eat?

Part of the problem is certainly the historical relationship between medical practice and the pharmaceutical industry. Doctors have the power to prescribe; they control distribution of the magic pills. It is a heady entitlement and the public wants the most "advanced treatment" regardless of effectiveness or even risk. This is high-tech, futuristic control of body chemistry. Changes in diet are not sexy, they sound mundane, tiresome, and boring. By focusing on treatment and avoiding prevention, the incidence of disease increases and the management of symptoms becomes more costly.

In America, just about 18 percent of the GNP is spent on health care; in the UK, the figure is 9.6 percent. Yet in an exhaustive survey done by the United Nations and published in 2000, America only ranked thirty-seventh out of 190 countries, and the UK ranked eighteenth. Something is seriously wrong, and money isn't fixing it. One problem is that the growing demands and increased complexity of treatment creates an environment where mistakes are unavoidable.

A 2013 report from the Institute of Medicine reported that there are 440,000 preventable deaths from medical errors annually in America. That makes medical error the third leading cause of death following heart disease and cancer. Be careful of hospitals; people die in there.

The focus of activity at the crash site is the prescription of pills. Every complaint, real or imagined, requires medication. Driven by pressure from the pharmaceutical industry and a cultural belief in the power of the pill, the abuse of prescriptive drugs grows yearly. An estimated forty-eight million Americans have abused prescription drugs (nearly 20 percent of the US population). Deaths by prescription drugs are more common than deaths by car accidents in America and far outstrip deaths by illegal drugs. Disturbingly, the nonmedical use of prescription drugs has been rising steadily for adolescents, particularly prescription pain relievers, anti-anxiety medications, stimulants, and steroids.

ANY PILL WILL DO

Sometimes doctors prescribe drugs under pressure from a misguided patient just to get them out of the office. There is ample research that shows that heart disease can be managed and even reversed through simple changes in lifestyle, and yet people are willing and eager to take dangerous drugs to offset the symptoms. The rate of diabetes in teens skyrockets; we know the cause, and yet the problem "needs more study." The long-term and combined effects of our romance with drugs are making us sicker. Antibiotics are a perfect example.

Antibiotics

Antibiotics first arrived on the medical scene in 1932. They were the first medicines labeled "wonder drugs." The introduction of the sulfa drugs meant the US mortality rate from pneumonia dropped from 0.20 percent each year to 0.05 percent by 1939. This was indeed a wonderful treatment and saved many lives. Penicillin (introduced a few years later) provided a broader spectrum of activity, and it had fewer side effects. Streptomycin, discovered in 1942, was the first effective drug against tuberculosis and came to be the best known of a long series of important antibiotics. The root causes of the diseases treated were lost in the celebrations.

Tuberculosis can be directly traced to individual and social behavior. This was also the case with whooping cough, pneumonia, and other diseases of poverty. They originate in crowded and unhygienic environments where malnutrition is common. When we were able to cure the illnesses with antibiotics, we stopped focusing on cleaning up the slums and the provision of healthy food.

The Negative Impact of Antibiotics

Antibiotics are specifically designed to kill microorganisms, but it is almost impossible to target a single species of the little critters. Antibiotics are literally "anti-life." We may kill the bacteria we want to kill, but we also kill or damage beneficial bacteria and mutate harmful ones. It is the medical equivalent of carpet bombing a whole population to kill one terrorist.

As antibiotic use increases, bacteria adapt to them and become resistant. A report by the Centers for Disease Control and Prevention stated that at least two million people annually "acquire serious infections with bacteria that are resistant to one or more of the antibiotics designed to treat those infections." at least twenty-three thousand people die annually in America from antibiotic-resistant infections.

The human body is home to about 100 trillion microbes. They inhabit every part of the body from the eyelash to the gut. They perform essential tasks in protecting us from potential pathogens. Many of these microorganisms are crucial to our digestive system. They form the microbiome in our gut which is the key to efficient metabolism, fine-tuning immune response, and even synthesize some vitamins.

It seems clear that the overuse of antibiotics is having a negative impact on many indigenous organisms in the human gut. These microbes have established a commensal (mutually beneficial) relationship with their human hosts. Their disappearance—under the onslaught of antibiotics and the modern diet—seems to promote conditions such as obesity and asthma. The use of antibiotics dramatically alters digestive function. Think of the common side effects of nausea and diarrhea. This is part of a vicious cycle: our diet makes us more prone to disease, and then we take drugs that hamper digestion and compromise immune function. Talk about throwing the baby out with the bath-water.

A recent study in the British National Health Service found that nine out of ten general practitioners in the UK feel pressurized by their patients to prescribe antibiotics. Around 97 percent of these patients are prescribed antibiotics *regardless of their illness*. When the National Institute for Health and Care Excellence (NICE) suggested that doctors who overprescribe be censured, doctors were upset.

"These can be very difficult and stressful conversations for GPs to have," said Dr. Tim Ballard, vice chair of the Royal College of GPs. "We need a societal change in attitudes towards the use of antibiotics."

We might ask the doctor who he expects to drive this societal change. If not doctors, then who will take the lead? Surely the medical profession should have the courage to tell an unpopular truth when it protects health? The problem's root causes (lifestyle or social issues) are not seen as medical issues unless they threaten medical authority.

MEDICAL FAITH

Taking medication is a huge act of faith. Some drugs are useful. Some are not. The relationship between the healer and the patient has always been one of simple belief. We believe that the healer knows about invisible forces and knows how to control them. It doesn't matter if the healer is a shaman on the Mongolian tundra, a wise woman herbalist in the forests of ancient Europe, or a doctor in modern America.

That does not mean that the doctor is practicing voodoo, it simply means that there is often a suspension of critical thinking on the part of the patient. Doctors may unwittingly support and encourage this mindset. It is not healthy. We need to be able to ask questions and get straight answers from our doctors.

Did you ever notice that nurses or receptionists always say how lucky you are, that your doctor is the best in his or her field? It is an infantile bond but also disempowering to the one seeking help. We are uneducated about health, and the doctor is unlikely to have the time (or perhaps the inclination) to educate us. It's busy at the crash site. They simply want to treat us and move on. So we continue thinking that we must hand over the care of our health to our doctor, and that they know what they are doing.

To increase the drama, disease is generally described as an enemy. Invisible and mysterious adversaries surround us and we need to fight back. We are "fighting" heart disease, we are "battling" cancer, and we will "conquer" diabetes. Who or what are we fighting? As long as the enemy is concealed behind a cloak of mystery, we can leave the battle up to the wizards and hope for the best. In order to discover the culprit, all that we need is a mirror. Our major antagonist is hiding in clear sight. We like to think that responsibility for our illnesses lies outside us. If my illness is caused by a virus, bacteria, or genetics, then I am faultless. But change my daily habits? Surely not! It can't be that simple. We seem willing to suffer any amount of pain or loss of dignity to avoid personal action.

A BAD REACTION

Increased drug use has led to a proliferation of "side effects" that are often more extreme and life-threatening than the condition being treated. Consider the drug Armodafinil (marketed in America as Nuvigil and manufactured by Cephalon Inc.). Armodafinil is used to treat daytime sleepiness caused by obstructive sleep disorder, or shift work disorder (only recently discovered, this ailment used to be called "not getting enough sleep"). It is also used as adjunctive therapy for disruptive breathing patterns during sleep (obstructive sleep apnea-hypopnea syndrome). The side effects of Armodafinil that require you to call your doctor include these:

- Blistering, burning, crusting, dryness, or flaking of the skin

- Burning, crawling, itching, numbness, prickling, "pins and needles," or tingling feelings

- Difficult or labored breathing

- Fast, irregular, pounding, or racing heartbeat or pulse

- Fever

- Frequent urination

- Increased volume of pale, diluted urine

- Itching, scaling, severe redness, soreness, or swelling of the skin or rash

- Severe and throbbing headache

- Shakiness in the legs, arms, hands, or feet

- Shortness of breath

- Tightness in the chest

- Trembling or shaking of the hands or feet

- Wheezing

Some side effects are signs of an overdose and require emergency treatment, such as the following:

- Anxiety
- Blurred vision
- Chest pain or discomfort
- Confusion about identity, place, and time
- Diarrhea
- Dry mouth
- Headache
- Hyperventilation
- Irritability
- Lightheadedness, dizziness, or fainting
- Nausea
- Nervousness
- Pounding in the ears
- Restlessness
- Seeing, hearing, or feeling things that are not there
- Sleeplessness
- Slow heartbeat
- Trouble falling asleep
- Unable to stay asleep
- Unusual tiredness or weakness

There are over twenty other side effects that include vomiting, loss of appetite, loss of interest or pleasure, trouble concentrating, and depression. This last group are said to be "less common" and may go away during treatment. The drug is, of course, FDA approved. I don't know about you, but I would seek a less brutal approach to "excessive daytime sleepiness"— something like a nap.

Criticizing the medical profession is not going to make anyone popular. We can criticize the "system" but not the doctors who operate in it. Everyone, including me, has a story of a loved one who has been helped by doctors. When someone dies while under medical treatment, or is destined to spend their life on medication that undermines the quality of their life, or is confined to a hospital or a care home to end their days hooked up to medical appliances, we are sad but resigned. We rarely ask if the treatment was essential, if the drugs were dangerous, or if there was an alternative treatment. We place our trust in those who supposedly know better and give up our own capacity for making decisions. Many years ago I was contacted by a woman who wanted to know more about the macrobiotic diet. She came to see me with her husband and told me she had been diagnosed with cancer and wanted to know about the possibility of improving her condition. After a long conversation and giving her a program, I asked the husband what kind of work he did. When he said he was an oncologist I almost fell out of my chair.

He told me that he and his wife had discussed her condition and he had received a second opinion on the diagnosis. She had been given only months to live. As a specialist he knew the suggested protocol for her cancer, the side effects, and the prognosis. They had decided to avoid the treatment because the cure rate was very low and the results of treatment would be both physically and psychologically devastating. They were both happy to have even months of quality time together till she passed away. She lived many months beyond her predicted death and enjoyed her family and clarity of mind. She was lucky she had a truly caring doctor in the house.

Prevention is better than cure, but the medical profession makes very little effort to prevent illness and is diligent in treatment at any cost, either emotional or physical. As long as doctors rely on symptomatic treatment with drugs and avoid a firm line on prevention, human health will deteriorate. The medical profession needs to concede that much of conventional treatment doesn't work, and diseases that are easily prevented continue to be treated with extreme measures.

A MEDICAL MIRAGE

One of my medical heroes was Dr. Robert Mendelsohn. Our first meeting was in the 1980s, at a conference on cancer and diet, sponsored by the East/West Foundation in Boston, Massachusetts. The foundation was a macrobiotic organization, and the event featured a panel of people who had cured themselves of serious diseases with the aid of the macrobiotic dietary approach. It was rare to see an orthodox physician at such an event at that time. Few were courageous enough to publicly endorse nonmedical approaches to healing, even if they knew they were effective.

After the testimonials, I was seated beside Mendelsohn for a panel discussion. While the introductions were being made, I whispered to him, "How did they persuade a doctor to come?" He smiled and said, "I'm a troublemaker, but I have good lawyers."

Mendelsohn was a pediatrician and had witnessed firsthand the ways that modern medicine was disempowering patients, especially women. He recognized the loss of choice and the damage that resulted from medical arrogance. His nationally syndicated column, the *People's Doctor*, had millions of fans. He was the national medical director of Project Head Start, chairman of the Medical Licensure Committee for the state of Illinois, an associate professor at the University of Illinois Medical School, and a director of Chicago's Michael Reese Hospital. He paved the way for people who questioned the old idea that "the doctor is always right." His attitudes are well summed up in his book *Confessions of a Medical Heretic:*

> When I was senior pediatric consultant to the Department of Mental Health in Illinois, I cut out a certain kind of operation that was being performed on mongoloid children with heart defects. The stated purpose of the operation was to improve oxygen supply to the brain. The real purpose, of course, was to improve the State's residency programs in cardiovascular surgery, because nothing beneficial happened to the brains of mongoloid children—and the surgeons knew that.
>
> The whole idea was absurd. It was also deadly since the operation had a fairly high mortality rate. Naturally, the university people were very upset when I cut out the operation. They couldn't figure out a better use for the mongoloid children, and besides, it was important to train people. In prepaid group practices where surgeons are paid a steady salary not tied to how many operations they perform, hysterectomies and tonsillectomies occur only about one-third as often as in fee-for-service situations.

THE BITTER PILL

Another huge problem in the medical system is the corrupt relationship between the medical profession and pharmaceutical companies, which effectively blocks the honest treatment of patients. Marcia Angell, a physician and longtime editor-in-chief of the *New England Medical Journal* (NEMJ), has caused quite a stir over the years with her ongoing critique of the relationship between the pharmaceutical industry and medical practice and research.

The FDA also relies increasingly upon fees and other payments from the pharmaceutical companies whose products the agency is supposed to regulate. This could contribute to the growing number of scandals in which the dangers of widely prescribed drugs have been discovered too late.

Last year, GlaxoSmithKline's diabetes drug Avandia was linked to thousands of heart attacks, and earlier in the decade, the company's antidepressant Paxil was discovered to exacerbate the risk of suicide in young people. Merck's painkiller Vioxx was also linked to thousands of heart disease deaths. In each case, the scientific literature gave little hint of these dangers. The companies have agreed to pay settlements in class-action lawsuits amounting to far less than the profits the drugs earned on the market. These precedents could be creating incentives for reduced vigilance concerning the side effects of prescription drugs in general.

The list of doctors and scientists who are repelled by the dishonesty that threads through medical practice and research grows longer every year. Dr. John Bailer, who spent twenty years on the staff of the National Cancer Institute and is also a former editor of its journal, publicly stated in a meeting of the American Association for the Advancement of Science:

My overall assessment is that the national cancer program must be judged a qualified failure. The five-year survival statistics of the American Cancer Society are very misleading. They now count things that are not cancer, and because we are able to diagnose at an earlier stage of the disease, patients falsely appear to live longer. Our whole cancer research in the past twenty years has been a total failure. More people over thirty are dying from cancer than ever before . . . More women with mild or benign diseases are being included in statistics and reported as being "cured." When government officials point to survival figures and say they are winning the war against cancer, they are using those survival rates improperly.

Wouldn't you think that all the knowledge about preventing disease would stimulate changes in attitude and action? But no. Medical arrogance delays any real change; medicine is "too big to fail." Doctors have basked in the warmth of civic esteem for so long that they are reluctant to admit that a radical shift is needed. Doctors would need to get behind reforms essential for promoting health or get out of the way and allow the reforms to happen.

A study published in the *American Journal of Clinical Nutrition* showed that the average medical student was given 23.9 hours of nutrition instruction. That's one day out of fifteen years. Nutrition, like the prevention of illness, gets pushed to the side in modern medical training (and, therefore, practice). Doctors don't know much about nutrition, but they act as if they do. I regularly hear from clients, students, and friends of doctors making absurd statements regarding diets and health. But we believe our doctors.

The relationship between disease and diet is well documented. According to the International Agency for Research in Cancer, over 80 percent of human cancer is caused by environmental factors. Those factors include smoking, diet, exposure to environmental toxins, and alcohol. In other words, they are avoidable causes.

The traffic in the cancer lane is steadily increasing, but where are the doctors pushing for change? Persuasion from doctors that patients (and society) change their ways is only a whisper. As medical historian Hans Ruesch says,

> Despite the general recognition that 80 percent of all cancers are caused by environmental influences, less than 10 percent of the (US) National Cancer Institute budget is given to environmental causes. And despite the recognition that the majority of environmental causes are linked to nutrition, less than 1 percent of the National Cancer Institute budget is devoted to nutrition studies. And even that small amount had to be forced on the Institute by a special amendment of the National Cancer Act in 1974.

The vast majority of doctors seem unwilling to make demands on politicians and business leaders to improve health in the most direct and effective ways. Could it be that there is a vested interest in keeping the sickness service running smoothly? Disease is big business. The corporate side of treating cancer is in a golden era. Spending on cancer medicines has hit a new milestone: US $100 billion in 2014 out of global sales of one trillion. Why would anyone be inspired to prevent a sickness that is such a cash cow? There is little doubt that the pharmaceutical industry is the driving force in forming medical policy.

NONCOMMUNICABLE DISEASE (NCD)

Some of you will undoubtedly think that I am being unfair to those doctors who are doing good work and trying to educate their patients; you may be right. I am also not addressing those situations where doctors are too busy fighting the rising tide of essential and/or emergency treatment to do the work of prevention. The responsibility of individuals to accept their part in creating their own health needs to be addressed as well.

The general public cannot claim total ignorance. For decades the connection between diet and disease has made its way through the ebb and flow of the news media. Cutting through the conflicting messages may be difficult but too few even make the effort. Change must come from a total reassessment of where the causes lie for our declining health and what should be done to reverse the trend. So let's look at the three major NCDs and how we deal with them, starting with heart disease.

Heart Disease

Heart disease is the leading cause of death in men and women. For many years, men ranked first in terms of the incidence of heart disease, but women are catching up rapidly. We know the causes of heart disease. It is the one of the most preventable (and probably the most studied) of all the noncommunicable diseases. Studies over the last few decades prove that the two main causes of heart disease are smoking and diet. Thankfully, fewer smokers have resulted in lower rates of heart disease, but we have done almost nothing to address diet and heart disease.

- About 600,000 people die of heart disease in the United States every year. That's one in every four deaths.

- Heart disease is the leading cause of death for both men and women. More than half of the deaths due to heart disease in 2009 were men.

- Coronary heart disease is the most common type of heart disease, killing nearly 380,000 people annually.

- Every year, about 720,000 Americans have a heart attack. Of these, 515,000 are a first heart attack, and 205,000 happen in people who have already had a heart attack.

- Coronary heart disease alone costs the United States $108.9 billion each year. This includes the cost of health-care services, medications, and lost productivity. You could put over 700,000 students through college for four years with that amount of money.

The World Heart Foundation says,

The role of diet is crucial in the development and prevention of cardiovascular disease. Diet is one of the key things you can change that will impact all other cardiovascular risk factors.

Comparisons between a diet low in saturated fats, with plenty of fresh fruit and vegetables, and the typical diet of someone living in the developed world show that in the former there is a 73 percent reduction in the risk of new major cardiac events.

Diabetes

The number of adults in the US with diabetes has tripled between 1980 and 2011. It is the seventh leading cause of death in America. Worldwide, the number of adults with diabetes will rise from 285 million in 2010 to 439 million in the year 2030.

We know a lot about diabetes. For instance, we know that type 2 diabetes accounts for between 90 percent and 95 percent of diagnosed adult cases. We are seeing more and more adolescents presenting with symptoms of type 2 diabetes. We know that diabetes contributes to heart disease, blindness, and is the main cause of kidney failure and lower limb amputation. It causes over 73,000 amputations a year (that's 1,400 a week). "Management" of the disease does not prevent these complications. It simply delays them. Yet we also know that diabetes is not only preventable, it is reversible.

Researchers at the University of Newcastle (UK) showed that using a low-calorie diet could reverse diabetes. It has also been shown that diabetics who had bariatric surgery and reduced their weight by 15 kg showed signs of recovery. Thousands of people using alternative health care have experienced a complete reversal of type 2 diabetes.

Naveed Sattar, professor of metabolic medicine at the University of Glasgow, is one of the UK's leading diabetes researchers. He sees successful management of type 2 diabetes as a curse. "It is moving us away from serious attempts to cure the problem. We're getting pretty good at keeping people alive longer," he says. "And we're seeing more and more obese younger people going on to tablets even earlier. That means the population living with diabetes is rising." There is too much focus on management and not enough on prevention.

My own experience with people with type 2 diabetes is that those given a good diet and good exercise program always see a dramatic improvement in their condition within two or three weeks. Most of them have reduced or completely come off their medication and are free of the disease. These results are not unusual. Many doctors and alternative practitioners in Europe and America see these kinds of results using a plant-based diet.

Cancer

When medical people talk about cancer they focus on the survival rates, and they can give us good news. Survival from cancer has doubled over the past forty years, the death rates have fallen and over half of all patients now survive at least ten years. We can now keep people alive with the disease. What we hear less regularly is that the occurrence of cancer is continually rising.

It is predicted there will be 23.6 million new cancer cases worldwide each year by 2030, recent trends in incidence of major cancers and population growth are seen globally in the future. This is 68 percent more cases than in 2012, with slightly larger growth in low and medium HDI *[Human Development Index]* countries (66 percent more cases in 2030 than 2012) than in high and very high HDI countries (56 percent more cases in 2030 than 2012).

The following figures are from a study that analyzed statistics from 1975 to 1994 on the incidence of all cancers. The findings indicated that while the incidence of some cancers was decreasing, others were rising at an alarming rate. (The most dramatic decline was in cases of lung cancer, as a result of fewer people smoking.) There are some shocking figures in the report.

- A contemporary black woman's risk of breast cancer is 54 percent greater than was her mother's at the same age. A white woman's risk is 41 percent greater than her mother's.

- Men today are three or four times more likely to be diagnosed with prostate cancer than their fathers.

- Excluding cancers linked to smoking, or where trends are confounded by changes in diagnostic procedure (breast and prostate), relative to the previous generation, rates increased on average 13 percent in black women, 52 percent in white men, and 67 percent in black men. There was little change in white women.

- For non-Hodgkin's lymphoma, which was analyzed separately, the rates today relative to those twenty-five years ago have almost doubled in white women, nearly tripled in black women, more than tripled in white men, and more than quadrupled in black men.

We can start looking at preventing cancer. Or we can continue to find ways to try and extend our lives with drugs by six months, eight months, or even some years. This "living with the disease" usually means that the quality of life is extremely compromised.

Numerous studies from the past thirty years link breast cancer to dairy food. Prostate cancer has been linked with the consumption of animal foods, particularly grilled meat. But this is not a popular message for media to cover, and it doesn't go down too well with food producers or pharmaceutical companies either.

Organized medicine presents its successes to us with a flourish and brushes its' unfortunate failures under the carpet. If medicine were really successful in creating health, we would need fewer hospitals, and medical services would not labor under stress.

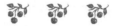

We are not condemned to continue feeding the money machines that both medicine and nutrition have become. There are things we can do to get out of this mess. We could stringently investigate the pharmaceutical industry's hold on the health-care industry. We could independently test all drugs and assess their value. We could insist that all approaches by the pharmaceutical lobbies to physicians and politicians are transparent. (Pharmaceutical lobbies have spent over $2.3 billion to directly influence lawmakers, and $183 million on political contributions since 1998.) The industry invested over $10 million on the 2016 American elections and make no mistake, it is an investment with expected huge returns.

The debates in health care seem to always revolve around who will pay, not what's being sold. It makes no difference if a single payer or an insurance company pays the bill if nothing is done to relieve the need for treatment.

Diet is a major cause of disease. This is good news because we can change our diet pretty easily. In the late 1960s, a revolution was brewing that challenged medical and nutritional mythologies, and it wasn't generated from within the ivory towers of universities. A rebellious public was asking increasingly difficult questions that generated some stunning changes that are discussed in the next chapter.

4

$\mathcal{Q}$uestioning Authority

Social change does not happen in a vacuum. It may take decades of debate or unrest before a new idea moves from "outsider belief" into the mainstream. Nutrition has been particularly resistant to change. It is primarily commercial priorities that apply the brakes. It has taken decades of pressure for the official voices of nutrition to be dragged, kicking and screaming, into accepting its own science. A growing interest in nutrition was influenced greatly by several shifts in public attitudes about health care in general. Some of these shifts helped redefine the role of the individual in their own health care and the right of the public to question medical authority.

Most of these shifts originated in the grass roots of society and some attitudes that have existed for hundreds of years. The notion of self-determination in health-care choices has been with us since the first days of the American republic. It was seen as a natural expression of the American experiment. During the first Constitutional Convention, Dr. Benjamin Rush, one of the Constitution signatories, made this prophesy:

> The Constitution of this Republic should make special provision for medical freedom. To restrict the art of healing to one class will constitute the Bastille of medical science. All such laws are un-American and despotic. Unless we put medical freedom into the Constitution, the time will come when medicine will organize into an undercover dictatorship and force people who wish doctors and treatment of their own choice to submit to only what the dictating outfit offers.

THE EARLY DAYS

The public had a broad range of medical options for many years. The medicine of the frontier settlers, mostly herbs and tonics, had been supplemented by homeopathy, which was introduced in 1825. There was a clear distinction between the allopathic and homeopathic doctors. Those physicians who were outside of the allopathic circle were called "irregulars" (now many would be called alternative practitioners). The medicines that were being prescribed by the allopaths (the "regular" doctors) were a grab bag of toxic potions often based on mercury compounds. The "undercover dictatorship" that Rush predicted grew slowly with the urbanization of America.

The American Medical Association (AMA)

The American Medical Association (AMA) charged hefty fees to drug companies advertising in their journal, in exchange for the AMA "seal of approval." The drug companies didn't have to provide any drug research or prove effectiveness or safety. They just had to list the ingredients and buy ads in all the local and regional issues of the journal. The drug companies funneled massive amounts of money to the AMA, and gave the exclusive access to their drugs. The money created political power.

Homeopaths, osteopaths, chiropractors, herbalists, and anyone practicing "irregular" medicine were dismissed as quacks and frauds by the AMA publicity machine. Some of these accusations were true, but the very drugs the AMA distributed were also unproven and many were dangerous. The AMA insisted that other approaches were "unscientific." The hypocrisy was transparent.

In 1900, Mark Twain observed:

> The doctor's insane system has not only been permitted to continue its follies for ages, but has been protected by the State and made a close monopoly. It is an infamous thing, a crime against a freeman's proper right to choose his own assassin or his own method of defending his body against disease and death.

Unfortunately this "insane system" continues to exist today.

The Flexor Report

The nail in the coffin of alternative medicine was the 1906 Flexner Report, sponsored by John D. Rockefeller. A survey of medical schools and practices, the report served as a guideline for legislation that would only license doctors trained in patented (manufactured) chemical-based drugs and surgery. The multimillionaires Rockefeller, J. P. Morgan, and Dale Carnegie profited greatly from this move, since they had purchased the huge German drug cartel IG Farben. The leverage that these industrialists had with politicians and government policy assured a monopoly to the AMA, which had previously existed only as a trade union.

Up until the 1950s, the AMA was still making money advertising products, including untested drugs, food products, and cigarettes that clamored for the implicit approval of this "scientific" body. Ads in the *JAMA* from the 1930s to the 1950s featured doctors claiming that "more doctors smoke Camels than any other brand" or that "ten months of scientific evidence shows that Chesterfield Cigarettes are more mild." As late as 1960, while the public commonly referred to cigarettes as "coffin nails" and the American Cancer Society had stated that the link between smoking and lung cancer had been proven "beyond a reasonable doubt," only one-third of all US doctors believed that the case against cigarettes had been established. My own doctor when I was a child constantly smoked in his office.

WOMEN STORM THE BARRICADES

In the early 1960s, thalidomide had been prescribed to pregnant women for anxiety, morning sickness, or insomnia, mostly in Germany. The outcome was tragic and shocking. Ten thousand children worldwide were born with severe birth defects to the arms and legs. About 50 percent of these children died. The message was that the doctors' judgment could be wrong and that prescribed drugs could kill.

Many in the general public were beginning to doubt the infallibility of doctors, and many had never stopped their use of naturopaths, chiropractors, homeopaths, or herbalists. In 1966, Dr. Henry Beecher wrote a groundbreaking article in the *New England Journal of Medicine* detailing his study of a hundred experiments conducted on patients by medical researchers. He found that twenty-two of these experiments were extremely dangerous for the patients. Some of these were organized in teaching hospitals, the US armed forces, and many with the approval of state boards of mental health. Some of these studies were conducted on the illiterate and patients in mental hospitals with dangerous substances to observe the results. The victims of these studies were being used as lab rats. These were highly questionable procedures without any known benefit to the patients and no informed consent.

Prescribing Sedatives on the Rise

There were worries by many health professionals that the increased prescriptions for sedatives were undermining public health. Valium hit the marketplace in 1963 and became the most prescribed drug in history. While the children of the middle classes were smoking pot and discovering LSD, their parents were becoming addicted to psychoactive sedatives, tranquilizers, and stimulants.

Women, in particular, were becoming sensitive to the casual misogyny that was institutionalized in medical practice. Why were pregnancy and childbirth being approached as illnesses? Why were women being discouraged to breastfeed? And why were so many problems experienced only by women being treated by men? Of special interest were the antidepressants Miltown, Librium, and Valium (Mothers Little Helpers), which were frequently prescribed to women. The drugs were even promoted in ways that implied that they would facilitate the strengthening of male authority at home and help to "calm women down" in the office.

Breast Is Best

Benjamin Spock had inspired many women to question their doctor's advice in the late 1940s and '50s. His book, the *Common Sense Book of Baby and Child Care*, created many debates within medicine and in the public. Pediatricians routinely told mothers to feed their children according to a fixed schedule. Spock counselled them to disregard doctors' orders and rely on their own instincts. The message was well-received, and the book became a best seller. When I met with Spock several years before he passed away, he commented on how he wished he had known more about diet during his early years. The last edition of his famous book was published after his death. In it, he recommended a vegan macrobiotic diet for children after weaning.

By the end of World War II, most women bottle-fed their babies, as encouraged by their doctors. There was no scientific reason for this, but there were many commercial ones. Baby formula was big business but some women were not buying it. In 1956, two mothers who met at a picnic in Illinois joined together with some friends to form the La Leche League. They were frustrated by the lack of good information about breastfeeding. The La Leche League became a major source of health information for new mothers. This happened in spite of medical opinion. The baby-formula issue is a perfect example of medicine supporting bogus nutrition.

Henri Nestlé, a Swiss food manufacturer, invented his first baby formula in 1867. The powdered formula consisted of malt, cows' milk, sugar, and processed wheat flour; it was to be mixed with water. Early advertisements said that it would help your baby get big and strong and walk early. Hospitals gave away free samples with every birth, along with instructions on bottle-feeding.

Nestlé's success was followed by Carnation concentrated milk. It was claimed that the milk came from "contented cows." Mothers all over the world were being schooled in the mythology that female breast milk was inadequate nutrition for healthy babies, that a manufactured product was superior nutrition, and that the milk of a cow was essential for human health. This fable was driven by commercial forces, and it lives on today among the vast majority of mothers in Western society.

A Rise in Activism

Dr. Spock and the women of the La Leche League exemplify the activist tone growing in the 1950s and '60s, questioning medical infallibility, highlighting patients' rights, and demanding transparency in medical treatment. An important discussion developed outside the medical and scientific community concerning self-determination in matters of personal health. A primary issue was the common practice of "benevolent deception," whereby physicians withhold information they feel might be detrimental to a patient's prognosis.

This principle was stated clearly in the AMA's original Code of Medical Ethics that advised, "The obedience of a patient to the prescriptions of his physician should be prompt and implicit. [The patient] should never permit his own crude opinions as to their fitness to influence his attention to them." It is a straightforward claim that the ethics of society at large are secondary to scientific orthodoxy. (It is a claim that still creates confusion today and is actively used to undermine dissent.) The idea that "doctor knows best" needed revision, and more of those "crude opinions" were being voiced.

Unsurprisingly, women were at the forefront of this new questioning of health care. Women bore the brunt of the increasing medicalization of society. In 1965, the rate of C-section births was 4.5 percent on the rise (it would reach 22.7 percent in 1985). In the twentieth century, childbirth in the developed world moved from the home to the hospital. Home birth rates fell to around 1 percent in the United Sates by the late 1970s. Some of this change was positive, but it was extreme measures indeed to treat every birth as a sickness that needed hospitalization.

One important force for change came with the 1970 publication of *Women and Their Bodies,* published by the *New England Free Press.* The booklet, the basis of a health course, was produced by twelve feminist activists from the Boston area. It dealt with issues such as "The Power and Role of Doctors" and "The Profit Motive in Health Care." One of the book's purposes was to create informed patients who would be empowered to deal with the health-care system. The book was expanded and republished in 1971 as *Our Bodies Ourselves* and became an instant best seller. It has sold over four million copies and been translated into twenty-nine languages.

Awareness of the potential abuses of medical authority was driving changes in the practice of medicine. There was progress in the treatment of women's health and in medical transparency. Patients' rights became a serious issue, which led to greater informed consent and client education. Unfortunately, the death grip of the pharmaceutical industry was not affected in any way, nor was the focus on treatment at the expense of prevention.

If medicine would not come to the rescue, then perhaps nutritionists would take up the challenge of disease prevention. Compelling nutritional studies pointed to the role of diet in heart disease and cancer. These never seemed to have any effect on public health policy, but the public was starting to wonder about the safety of their food.

EPIDEMIOLOGICAL INSIGHT

Study after study during the 1960s and '70s illustrated the dangers of the American diet and stirred arguments that still rage on today. The changes in nutrition were in some ways more fundamental and dramatic than the shifts in medicine regarding public health. Consumers were questioning orthodox nutritional science and beginning to demand more "natural" and unadulterated food. Those seeking a healthy diet were marching to their own drum. This new dietary trend was powerful, but it was not without problems.

Nutritional Science

Nutritional science is plagued with dilemmas that separate it from many other branches of scientific inquiry. The usual rule of science is replication of studies. You run an experiment and then you run it again, to ensure that the results are the same. However, no one yet has isolated a population of humans—fed them the same diet, confined them to exactly the same environment, and then performed the autopsies that might prove how the diet affected their health.

Studies on the effect of specific nutrients are done in laboratories on test animals, or in petri dishes. But the animals and the petri dishes can't replicate human life, or the diversity of digestive microbes in the human gut, or any of the environmental factors that affect what we eat and how it nourishes us. While these studies are of interest, they cannot replicate the relationships between diet and health. They can only offer generalizations.

Observational Studies

Many believe epidemiology offers better insight. Epidemiology produces observational studies that deal with actual humans going about their daily lives. If the sample is large enough and diverse influences are taken into account, extremely interesting data can emerge. Studying a particular ethnic population, who migrate to a new society, could present some relevant insight, particularly if some people adapt their diet to the new cultural norm and some don't. A marked change in the health of those who adapt to the new diet (in terms of diseases) could be significant. Here's a case in point.

Japanese women, for decades, had a much lower rate of breast cancer than American women. It was noted in several studies that Japanese women who moved to the United States and adopted an American diet soon had the same incidence of the disease as American women. Those who continued with the Japanese diets did not. Therefore, differences in cancer risk between the US and Japan were not due to genetics. The critical difference was in the amount of fat eaten, particularly animal fat. Studies of this kind have become an important reference point in modern nutritional thinking.

RELATIONSHIP BETWEEN DIET AND DISEASE

In 1956, the US Public Health Service funded the Seven Countries Study to investigate the relationship between diet and cardiovascular disease. This was the first epidemiological study to compare habits and disease patterns in seven different countries: Finland, Italy, Japan, Netherlands, Yugoslavia, Greece, and the United States. The study was directed by Ancel Keys, who had identified a correlation between high cholesterol and cardiovascular disease in a group of American businessmen.

The program has continued for over fifty years, and it shows findings similar to those discovered by the Framingham Heart Study, the Nurses' Health Study, and countless other investigations. The results may not sound too radical to us now. Smoking and America's high-fat diet were primary contributors to the rising cholesterol levels that contributed to coronary heart disease, obesity, and increases in cancer deaths. Conversely, exercise and diets rich in plant foods and fiber provided protection against disease.

The Seven Countries Study would eventually lead to the creation of the Mediterranean Diet (which was not, in fact, specific to any country but a general reflection of eating patterns). The diet was high in fruits, whole grains, nuts, legumes, olive oil, and vegetables, and it was low in animal fats, with some fish, but little dairy or meat. It was certainly an improvement as far as it went, but nutritional infighting was to create just the right amount of confusion to prevent consensus.

The US Senate created the Select Committee on Nutrition and Human Needs in 1968. The intent of the committee was to investigate the issue of hunger among the old, the poor, and the young. After some years, they began to focus also on the relationship between diet and disease. Inspired by the Seven Countries Study, they encouraged the National Institutes of Health to support further research.

Attacks From the Food Industry

On release of the committee's report, its findings were immediately attacked by the food industry. The suggestion that people should reduce their consumption of meat, eggs, and foods high in fat, sugar, and salt (the basis of the American diet) was considered heresy. The food industry was outraged. (You don't want the government telling people not to buy your products, even if they are dangerous.) In 1968, a congressional committee was formed under the leadership of Senator George McGovern. The Senate Committee was to review the science and make suggestions regarding the American diet.

In 1977, the proposal of Dietary Guidelines drew the wrath of the meat industry, who recommended the committee withdraw the guidelines and issue a corrected report. They especially didn't like a suggestion to "decrease meat consumption to lower saturated fat intake."

Kansas senator Robert Dole suggested changing *"decrease* consumption of meat" to "increase consumption of *lean* meat."

"Would that taste better to you?" he asked the president of the cattlemen's association.

"Decrease is a bad word, Senator," was the reply.

In the end, the bottom-line considerations won the day. A revised edition of the report was published later that year, and the phrase "reduce consumption of meat" was changed to "choose meats, poultry, and fish that will reduce saturated fat intake." Throughout the report, any suggestion to reduce consumption of a food was rephrased to encourage the consumer to use the food wisely "as part of a healthy

diet." The original report was watered down to benefit the food producers; issues of health were sidelined.

It wasn't long before the Senate Committee on Nutrition and Human
Needs was disbanded. The responsibility of nutrition guidelines was
passed to the Department of Agriculture, a government agency with the
closest ties to the producers of food.

This is still common. In January 2016, the Washington-based non-
profit Physicians Committee for Responsible Medicine filed a lawsuit
against Agriculture secretary Tom Vilsack and Sylvia Mathews Burwell,
secretary of Health and Human Services. The suit seeks to reinstate
a dietary recommendation on limiting cholesterol, which had been
omitted from the 2016 publication of the report in response to industry
pressure.

Nutritional Debates

Battles within the field of nutritional science are bad for the general
public. Individual nutritionists and doctors have put their own spin on
the avalanche of studies released over the past decades. While some
commentary was serious and considered, much was simple, unscientific
opinion published in popular magazines.

With portion sizes increasing yearly and food technology creating
new products that cater to every possible sensory impulse, nutritional
clarity is a real challenge. The official default "be moderate" approach
says that the food is fine; just stop being greedy.

Nutritional debate always seems to prompt a return to the lab to
find the micro-scoundrel—the elusive outlaw nutrient—that causes the
problems. After all, it's all about the chemistry. Too much fat in the
diet? Remove some fat from milk and call it "low fat." Replace butter
with margarine and say that it's "heart healthy." Replace sugar with
chemicals and call it "low calorie." Food science was on a roll—food
was being disassembled, reformed, and "enhanced," supposedly for
better health. Yet the rates of obesity and food-related disease kept
creeping upward.

The student free speech, civil rights, and anti-war movements of the
1960s had a popular motto: Question Authority. People understood that
previously sacrosanct institutions, such as politics, religion, and even

science, often had an agenda that was counter to the public good. The natural foods movement expressed this spirit of social rebellion against nutritional dogma.

A generation that had been influenced by the writing of Rachel Carson was aware of the growing use of artificial pesticides, and herbicides in agriculture. If toxic chemicals in the environment were poisoning birds and other wildlife, what would they do to humans?

MACROBIOTICS AND FOOD ACTIVISM

The book that my friends and I used as our travel guide into the world of healthy eating was *Zen Macrobiotics* by a Japanese philosopher named George Oshawa. Oshawa appealed to his younger audience through a combination of Eastern spiritual concepts, environmental sensibility, and a unique vision of how healthy people could create a healthy world.

Oshawa applied his particular version of Chinese medical theory to nutrition. He was part of a Japanese tradition of "food doctors" that stretched back to the 1600s. His inspiration was his own recovery from tuberculosis, which came about through using a way of eating that he labeled "macrobiotics." By the late nineteenth century, this branch of Far Eastern medicine was attempting to combine the understanding of folk traditions with Western science.

After his death, Oshawa's students continued his work. Many had moved to other countries to teach his philosophy. The most prominent of these was Michio Kushi, who had moved to America and had begun teaching in the 1950s. Kushi and his wife, Aveline, would prove to be two of the most influential (although barely acknowledged) people in the birth of the modern natural foods movement in America.

I traveled to Boston, Massachusetts, in 1967 to learn more about this dietary approach and the macrobiotic philosophy behind it. I had already experienced the benefits of dietary change and observed its effect on many friends. I was driven by curiosity and those two questions that my experience with my doctor had conjured up: "Why was my doctor so antagonistic regarding my diet?" and "How did the ancient doctor/philosophers in the Far East figure out the principles of a healthy diet without any technology?"

Kushi gave classes in the basement of the historic Arlington Street Church by the Boston Commons. Every week, a group of twenty to fifty people would gather and listen to him speak about a wide range of issues. His unique gift was the ability to illustrate the connections between seemingly different areas of study. A lecture on history might end up with a discussion on farming methods. Connections might be made between the physical form of a plant and its medicinal uses. There was always something about diet and health, but the reference point was not about nutrients—it was about our relationship to the environment and our awareness of our actions. Kushi was presenting a new vision of health care that was not governed by established medicine or nutrition but by the power of personal responsibility, the development of sensitivity to biological change, and self-generated healing.

It was the invasion of Asian ideas that animated much of the interest in a healthy diet. Chinese medicine, Japanese Folk Medicine, and Indian Ayurvedic medicine were not only cultural oddities but were introducing new ways of understanding health. Indian yogis were introducing yoga and Indian-inspired vegetarian food to the West, and Japanese teachers were promoting their unique ways of classifying foods, Zen meditation, and the principles of Chinese medicine.

The idea of the "body as a temple" was making a comeback after many centuries of virtual slumber. The concept of peaceful living linked itself naturally to physical health, and to the avoidance of cruelty to animals, and it seemed to fit the growing movement toward living in harmony with nature.

The macrobiotic movement was not founded on standard nutritional information but on ecological principles. Attention was paid to eating simple, unprocessed, natural food and being aware of the influence of seasonal changes, the specific properties of the food eaten, the effects of the preparation/cooking of the food, and individual needs. The focus was to become sensitive to the relationship between diet and daily well-being.

THE JUNK FOOD ALTERNATIVE

Erewhon Trading Company, the macrobiotic shop in Boston, became a template for an explosion of small shops, stores, and community co-ops.

The focus was consumer education. We put small tear-off information sheets next to most products. People could find out exactly where the food came from (and, in most cases, who grew it). They could learn why the oils were "cold-pressed" and not chemically extracted, and why there was no sugar in the dessert items. We trusted that if consumers were informed, they would make the right choices. In the *History of Erewhon*, William Shurtleff writes:

> The modern natural foods movement, which started as a macrobiotic foods movement in the mid-1960s, has continued until the present. It began with the idea of changing the existing health-food business into something new and different—the natural foods business. Young men and women who came of age during the period from 1960 to 1980 founded it.
>
> Theirs was a positive message. They wanted to grow and process foods naturally, and to make them widely available in a way that would attract people to an alternative that was good for the body and for the planet; by contrast, previous food movements had generally motivated people to avoid certain foods out of fear.
>
> These young people, most of whom considered themselves part of the counterculture, decided to try to create a new food system. Some started companies to make new foods (from whole-grain breads and pastries to tofu and miso). Hundreds (eventually thousands) of others started new natural foods stores—which (for the first 10 to 15 years) sold many foods unpackaged in bulk and would not sell meat, refined foods, or foods containing sugar or chemical additives, pills, alcohol, or tobacco.

In response, the traditional nutritional community tried to sow fear. Our old friend Dr. Fredrick Stare wrote an article in the *Reader's Digest* called "The Diet That's Killing Our Kids," and doctors warned of an epidemic of nutritional deficiency. But we didn't die, we weren't deficient, and we didn't give up. Good food was on the move.

In 1971, the author and social activist Frances Moore-Lappe published *Diet for a Small Planet*. The book addressed the issue of world hunger and pointed to the waste of food involved by feeding nutritious crops to animals instead of to humans. Many of us had been exposed to this idea in macrobiotics by Oshawa's version of the food economics of

Mahatma Gandhi. This vision was best stated as "There is enough for everyone's need but not everyone's greed." The social issues of world hunger, food distribution, and the efficacy of vegetable protein came racing into the food debate.

While the epidemiological studies showing the harmful effects of the American diet were being ineffectually debated by academics, the food industry, and politicians, the natural food movement was creating a vibrant and empowering social awareness of the power of food. By 1987, John Robbins's book *Diet for a New America*—which discussed vegetarianism, factory farming, and animal rights—became the go-to reference book for people interested in dietary reform. Meanwhile, the thousands of small shops and community co-ops demonstrated the commercial success of the natural foods revolution.

As the new natural foods stores became successful, they birthed a new wave of "healthy" retailers. These new stores presented a bit of the homey ambiance of the earlier food shops but played with clever marketing and less attention to quality. They carried a wider range of products and presented foods in a way that supermarket shoppers could understand.

Eventually, the lines between an upscale food emporium and a natural foods store became blurred. They became food boutiques. A different breed of customers was drawn into the new stores. These new consumers were often motivated by general fitness, concerns of aging, perceived food quality, and sometimes by a trendy exclusivity. There was little that distinguished affluent supermarkets and natural foods outlets. The vital issues of environmental impact of the foods or issues of social justice were used as marketing tools and did not drive serious action in the stores. The major growth in products was supplements, snack foods, cosmetics, and vegetarian/vegan products that mimicked familiar animal foods. Products such as non-dairy cheese, plant and seed milks, and mock meats flourished.

Nowadays, many popular "natural" chain stores use the same advertising approach as the conventional food trade. Consumers often feel the products are more powerful than they are in fact. Product labelling has become a serious issue. Ingredients such as "refined cane juice" (sugar), "agave" (fructose and sugar), or "coconut sweetener" (actually made from the sap of the coconut palm, with little difference between it and cane sugar) sound exotic. They might even sound healthy. But they're not. As John Yudkin said in reference to the difference between brown and white sugar, "It's the difference between a man standing naked and a man standing naked wearing a necktie."

SUPER FOODS

The focus of nutritional science on micronutrients has created a Tower of Babel. Individual nutrients are sought out to justify the use or avoidance of particular foods. "Superfoods" are discovered monthly. The suspected benefits of specific nutrients found in a food are often used to validate its use regardless of the value as part of a healthy diet. The world of the superfoods is an exotic exercise in marketing. It is an approach that caters to fears of deficiencies where there are none and devotion to the magical properties of the miracle food.

When I was growing up, there was an avocado tree near our house. Little did I know that avocados could cure cancer. But based on a study done by a real, live scientist at the University of Waterloo in Canada, a single fat in avocados combats acute myeloid leukemia by attacking stem cells. The study does not say that eating avocados will cure or even prevent cancer, but that doesn't stop extravagant claims or newspaper headlines.

I have nothing against avocados. Who doesn't like a bit of guacamole once in a while? But does eating avocados decrease cancer risk? It doesn't seem to. You would have to eat several pounds of them to get significant amounts of that single fat anyway. But then if the avocados don't work, you could always try coconuts!

Coconut oil, coconut butter, and all things coconut have been a huge boon to the coconut growers and processors over the past few years. The oil gained popularity in the 1990s as a vegetable oil that mimics some of the qualities of butter in making baked products. It is claimed that it has almost magical powers in healing cancers, candida, herpes, HIV, and baldness. It makes your skin younger, protects against heart disease, and helps you lose weight. Sounds like a winner—until you try to find any true studies to back up the claims. In fact, if we were to refer to science only, we might want to look at the report from Science and the Public Interest that laid down a detailed critique of the use of the oil in movie theater popcorn. It is 92 percent saturated fat. That is higher than lard. But if enough people wearing lab coats repeat something, it can easily be accepted as truth.

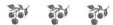

The overall effect of the AMA monopoly of health care in America best served the growth of the pharmaceutical industry. That industry not only dominates medical treatment but an important factor in understanding why more individuals do not embrace a healthy diet and lifestyle. It is an implicit encouragement of unhealthy habits, the results of which can be taken care of by drugs when they become painful or life threatening.

In the absence of medical modeling for nutritional and lifestyle changes, grassroots movements in the 1960's demonstrated the power of community education in healthy living. These movements still hold some social influence but are easily co-opted by commercial interests.

Most of the Natural Foods companies of that era have been bought out by large food corporations. Companies such as Coca Cola, Pepsico, Nestle, and General Foods, now control many of the producers of natural foods products. Whole Foods Markets are now controlled by Amazon. It is naive to believe that large corporations will maintain the integrity of the products. It is essential to dig deep into the research and practical experience of both the past and present "food rebels" to find the approach to nutrition that prevents disease and even healing. We will start the journey in the next chapter.

5

$\mathcal{T}$he Healing Kitchen

T
he cabal that consists of the pharmaceutical industry and medicine also includes those who grow and manufacture the food that starts the ball rolling. A handful of corporations dominate the world food supply that creates sickness and inequity. We need to escape this cycle of toxic causes that feed toxic treatment with only profit as a goal. Sickness is costly.

Finding a solution will take looking in some unexpected places. Both the ancient past and the avant-garde of modern nutrition offer practical solutions. Many of these solutions have been gathering attention over the last few decades and providing practical solutions that could not only reverse the tide of NCD's but also save money in the process.

According to the Integrated Benefits Institute, which represents major US employers and business coalitions, poor health costs the US economy $576 billion a year. About 39 percent of this (that's $227 billion) is from "lost productivity" due to absenteeism, or to poor performance from employees who are unwell.

Over the past decade, the issue of healthcare has been a political nightmare. There are accusations of socialist conspiracies and arguments about death panels for the elderly or the relative benefits of government healthcare as opposed to a free market. Regardless of how we deal with it, the cost of treating preventable disease is moving us toward financial disaster.

A 2009 study in the *American Journal of Medicine* revealed that medical expenses caused 62.1 percent of all bankruptcies in 2007. The strain on businesses is no different than on governments—everyone pays, directly or indirectly. Earlier I outlined some major diseases that are directly linked to diet. According to the Centers for Disease Control (CDC), seven of every ten American deaths are due to a chronic disease, and these diseases cost 75 percent of the nation's $2 trillion expense. Out of the CDC budget of $8.8 billion, only 9 percent goes to chronic disease prevention and health promotion. Of that 9 percent, less than 5 percent goes to areas of nutrition, physical activity, and obesity. Although we know about rising health costs and outdated health infrastructures, we are curiously reluctant to act.

The elephant in the room is prevention, which would eventually lead to questions of responsibility. So who do we name and shame for the rise of preventable food-caused disease? It seems that nobody is responsible for nutrition. They are just "doing their job": from the medical profession cleaning up the traffic crash to the food companies who just make the tasty treats the public wants to the politicians focused on the health of the stock market. Nutritionists are not even in the building—they are on chat shows telling people to "be moderate" and only eat 15 potato chips (the actual recommended serving) at a sitting. That leaves only the consumer, looking for guidance, lost at sea, bouncing from fad to fad or simply giving up and sinking in an ocean of junk food.

When many people share a habit, it becomes normalized. When smoking was common, very few people complained about smoke. In the 1950s, it was acceptable to smoke in almost every situation. Just look at movies from the 1940s and '50s; everyone was puffing away. It was even seen to be elegant. There were no consequences for driving after drinking—unless you caused an accident or were seen to be driving dangerously. Those behaviors were eventually acknowledged to be harmful, and social, economic, and government pressures were applied to curtail them.

Our resistance to changing unhealthy behavior is exacerbated by the illusion that if we experience pain or get sick, we can be patched up. This often involves drugs to make living in our damaged body more bearable.

The 2015 *Time* magazine cover story on painkillers pointed out that 9.4 million Americans take opioids for long-term pain, and the National

Institutes of Health estimates that 2.1 million are hooked. In 2017 there were 47,000 deaths due to opioids alone. Of the 220,400 overdose deaths registered in 2005, prescription drugs outnumbered street drugs by 6 percent.

AN OUNCE OF PREVENTION

Let's use obesity as our example, since it is so closely related to diet in the popular imagination. Obesity brings up a great deal of social conflict. Some see it as a disease or a genetic flaw and others as antisocial or as the outcome of a lack of self-esteem or self-control. It is increasingly prevalent despite its symptoms being in direct conflict with social body-image fashions.

Obesity increases inpatient and ambulatory healthcare costs by $395 per person per year (that's more than either smoking or problem drinking). In Scotland, £3.5 million was recently spent on new ambulances to carry the obese to the hospital. Some are angry that we have to pay these costs, but the causes of the obesity epidemic are still not addressed. The organization Diabetes UK has been lobbying the National Health Service to support bariatric surgery as a solution to the diabetes epidemic. Evidently, people are compelled to eat junk food, shrinking their stomachs will solve the problem.

> Diabetes UK supports the NICE recommendations on bariatric surgical and procedural interventions in the treatment of obese patients with type 2 diabetes. In particular, for those who have failed to lose weight through diet and lifestyle changes. This includes expediting assessment for bariatric surgery in recent onset type 2 diabetes.

Of course, the "diet and lifestyle changes" being used are absurd, and simply minor changes in the caloric values of food eaten and modest exercise are all that is required. The programs that they recommend have been shown not to work. Any serious student knows that the effect of these programs seldom produce any effect aside from paying a group of charity officials. Personal behavior is put forward as something that is completely governed by factors outside personal control.

Diet-related cancers and heart disease escape the degree of public scrutiny that obesity receives, despite overwhelming evidence that they are self-caused. Could it be because obesity is so visible and is seen as physically imperfect? Or that other maladies may be unnoticed until they become debilitating? Or is it simply because we have conditions that are inescapable and governed by fate? It is certainly not because they are less costly to the economy.

Heart disease and cancer are expensive. Heart disease in America costs $131.3 billion a year, and cancer expenses total $263.8 billion. Why is there so little outcry that we have to pay for other people's cancer and heart disease?

I invite you to do a little self-inventory right now and check out how that last paragraph affects you. The debate about healthcare invariably comes down to who pays. The answer is always that we all do one way or another. This is an important issue that strikes to the core of why we are unable to make meaningful dietary and health reforms. We feel compassion for anyone who is ill, of course we do. Responsibility is not about blame. We need to acknowledge the role of our collective and individual actions in creating such a high rate of preventable problems and then act on that knowledge.

Preventable disease is simply that—preventable. There is nothing mysterious about it. There are some genetic influences on cancer. Inherited mutations are thought to play a role in between 5 percent and 10 percent of all cancers, and they are only significant as tendencies, not certainties. The *Merriam-Webster* dictionary defines disease as:

A response to environmental factors (as malnutrition, industrial hazards, or climate), to specific infective agents (as worms, bacteria, or viruses), to inherent defects of the organism (as genetic anomalies), or to combinations of these factors.

Bacteria, viruses, and genetics are most people's favorite reasons for the cause of disease. They are mysterious and beyond control and yet the top six causes of death in Western society all have diet and lifestyle as primary risk factors. The "fight" against heart disease and the "war" on cancer excites our imagination. At one single event in Los Angeles, over $100 million was raised to "fight" cancer.

THE WAR ON CANCER

In 2015 in the UK, a series of spectacular television advertisements featured different determined women staring at the viewer and declaring "Watch out, cancer. We're coming to get you," or "Cancer, we're going to kick your butt." The angry, defiant words expressed the collective pain that so many experienced at losing loved ones. They, of course, were part of a fund-raising drive aimed at cancer research.

In his last State of the Union speech, President Obama appointed his vice president, Joe Biden, to lead the new "war against cancer." If we could send people into space, surely we could rally our best scientists to conquer cancer. It was a special moment when members of all parties could applaud the call to battle. If cancer was in the room, it didn't stand a chance.

Sadly, cancer research has been a gigantic waste of money that has only profited the pharmaceutical industry and charity executives. It is a con game. The pink ribbons and the celebrity testimonials all feed a powerful mythology supported by social fund-raising events, such as charity runs and (with no irony intended) bake sales. A little history about those pink ribbons is instructive.

The association with the ribbons was born out of Charlotte Haley's campaign to convince the National Cancer Institute (NCI) to increase the budget for cancer prevention. She gave peach-colored ribbons to those who supported her movement. She refused to commercialize her campaign, but Estée Lauder took her idea and simply changed the color of the ribbon to protect themselves from legal action. The Breast Cancer Awareness movement was born. Haley's desire to increase information on the prevention of cancer was put aside in favor of "awareness." Awareness is code for treatment and screening. Pink-ribbon products were a corporate bonanza and are a billion-dollar industry.

One of the sponsors of Breast Cancer Awareness Month and their pink ribbons is Zeneca Pharmaceuticals, the maker of tamoxifen. Tamoxifen is one of the major drugs used in cancer treatment, and Zeneca is owned by Imperial Chemical Industries. ICI also produces several products that are suspected carcinogens. They are joined in this dog-and-pony show by other sponsors, such as Monsanto, General Electric (makers of mammography machines), DuPont Chemical, and a broad selection of cosmetic companies, including Revlon and Mary Kay.

Cancer charities focus on the treatment of cancer rather than on prevention. There is scant attention to diet or lifestyle in National Cancer Institute literature and next to nothing on environmental hazards, such as pesticides. Prevention and early detection are confused in the public eye, but they are very different. Constant screening for cancer can be harmful since false-positive results are common and lead to unnecessary treatment. Charities help fund drug research that is then sold back to the patient or institution implementing the treatment—a boon for the drug industry.

A study done at Southampton University in the UK assessed claims that breast cancer screening could produce more harm than benefit. Their findings—that the screenings did, in fact, cause a net harm—were published in the *British Medical Journal*. In the words of the lead researcher, James Raflery:

> The default is to assume that screening must be good; catching something early must be good, but if a woman has an unnecessary mastectomy, or chemotherapy, or radiation, that's a tragedy. It is difficult to balance the gain of one life against two hundred false positives and ten unnecessary surgeries.

We should not place our faith in medicine without inquiring as to the facts. The attitudes and intentions of doctors and researchers are not universally honorable. Even those within the medical establishment question the quality and focus of research. Dr. Margaret Cuomo writes in her book *A World without Cancer*:

> Simply put, we have not adequately channeled our scientific know-how, funding, and energy into a full exploration of the one path certain to save lives: prevention. That it should become the ultimate goal of cancer research has been recognized since the war on cancer began. When I look at NCI's budget request for fiscal year 2012, I'm deeply disappointed, though past experience tells me I shouldn't be surprised. It is business as usual at the nation's foremost cancer research establishment. More than $2 billion is requested for basic research into the mechanism and causes of cancer. Another $1.3 billion is requested for treatment. Cancer prevention and control gets $232 million altogether. (Remarkably, in the very same budget

report, the NCI states, "Much of the progress against cancer in recent decades has stemmed from successes in the areas of prevention and control.")

MEDICAL FRAUD

Even the content of the research, when submitted and published, can be a problem. Dr. Marcia Angell—the long-serving editor in chief of the *New England Medical Journal*—shocked the medical community when she spoke out about the quality of research being produced.

> It is simply no longer possible to believe much of the clinical research that is published, or to rely on the judgment of trusted physicians or authoritative medical guidelines. I take no pleasure in this conclusion, which I reached slowly and reluctantly over my two decades as an editor of the *New England Journal of Medicine*.

Dr. Angell has written extensively on the false promises given by the drug companies and the medical profession. In an article for the *New York Review of Books*, she points to the many instances of fraud in research. The validity of these charges is backed up by the history of payments made for fraud by drug companies. The drug giants GlaxoSmithKline, Pfizer, Merck, Eli Lilly, and Abbott have all been convicted of fraud and forced to pay millions in fines. TAP Pharmaceuticals, for example, in 2001 pleaded guilty and agreed to pay $875 million to settle criminal and civil charges.

These millions in fines are of no consequence when compared to the profits generated—they are "the cost of doing business." The news of these crimes do not stay in the public eye for long. The fact that alternative or complementary medicine is condemned for "not being scientific" misses the irony of all the bad science that is out there.

The proportion of scientific research that is retracted due to fraud has increased tenfold since 1975, according to the most comprehensive analysis yet of "bad" research papers. The study for the National Academy of Sciences (PNAS) discovered that more than two-thirds of the retractions of biomedical and life sciences papers from the scientific record are due to misconduct by researchers rather than error. Of course, scientific misconduct and fraud directly impact areas such as medicine and health care.

Competition for research grants is intense, and the "right results" are desirable to both researcher and sponsor. In a 2009 meta-analysis of the prevalence of research misconduct, 2 percent of the scientists admitted to serious misconduct (including the fabrication of data) at least once, and up to 34 percent admitted questionable research practices. When asked about their colleagues' practices, the figures went through the roof. They accused colleagues of data falsification 14 percent of the time, and 72 percent for other questionable practices. With friends like these . . .

Medicine often claims that any non-science-based treatment is not valid. This quote by Dr. John G. Faughnan is typical:

> I think much of what is today called "alternative medicine" is, at best, effective placebo, and, at worst, fraud.

There is no question that fraud can and does exist in alternative treatment and should be exposed. Given the resistance to nonscientific approaches, it is important, then, that we assess the effectiveness of standard treatment as well. According to an article recently published in the *British Medical Journal* from 2003, the news is not great. Research into over three thousand treatments showed only 11 percent of the treatments were deemed beneficial, 24 percent were "likely" to be beneficial, 7 percent were a trade-off between benefit and harm, 5 percent were unlikely to be of benefit, 3 percent were likely to be ineffective or harmful, and a whopping 50 percent of the treatments were of unknown effectiveness. That means about 36 percent overall effectiveness or likely benefit. That certainly sounds like fraud to me.

This is in line with statements made by Dr. Allen Roses, vice president of genetics at GlaxoSmithKline, the world's second largest drug manufacturer. He says, "The vast majority of drugs (more than 90 percent) only work in 30 percent or 50 percent of the people." Some drug representatives were outraged, but many applauded his honesty.

Statements like this, and surveys that question treatment, are easy to take out of context. Some medications work with great consistency, and others do not. Extreme circumstances call for extreme measures, but the medical establishment treats every variation from the norm as extreme.

Even though approximately 2.2 million US hospital patients experience adverse drug reactions (ADRs) to prescribed medications yearly, we opt for the strongest possible treatment at the earliest possible moment. These should be last-ditch actions, but we prefer bombing to diplomacy.

A diplomatic approach would be to coax the natural healing mechanisms of the body to do their job. We know about the power of the immune system and the repair capacities of the body. We should attempt to harness these in the healing process rather than undermine and overwhelm them with antibiotics or suppress and disguise the symptoms. With what we know about the power of nutrition to impede or improve immune response, our daily diet becomes crucial. Natural healing—with nutrition at its core—is the leading edge of the nutrition revolution. The macrobiotic movement in America and Europe was an important part of that avant-garde.

MACROBIOTICS AND HEALING

When I began my studies with Michio Kushi, the focus was on personal development and ecological living. Conventional medicine did not at all consider that food could prevent or heal disease. Even making statements to that effect were dangerous. Government FDA investigators made unannounced appearances at macrobiotic food shops in New York and Boston to confiscate the books of George Oshawa.

Oshawa claimed sickness could be cured with food, and shops that were selling that food as well as the books were being accused of practicing medicine without a license. In a small Boston shop, Oshawa's books were hidden in the back of the store and were only available on request. They were not available to suited men with brown shoes and crew cuts.

Still, the movement toward understanding food as a therapeutic tool as well as for illness prevention was growing, largely as a response to the epidemiological studies mentioned earlier and the grassroots work of thousands of nonprofessional advocates of healthy eating. Studies like Ancel Keys's Minnesota Business and Professional Men Study and the Framingham Study fired the public imagination. People were asking questions like, "If changing your diet lowers your blood pressure and your cholesterol levels, why are drugs and surgeries being recommended?"

The growth of "alternative medicine" was largely driven by personal experiences. Many who had suffered from chronic pain or debilitating symptoms were reporting relief of symptoms through simple, mostly non-invasive therapies. There was a groundswell of interest in acupuncture, alternative nutritional approaches to healing, and mind/body techniques.

An increasing number of doctors were seeing unexpected cures and spontaneous remissions of disease. Interest was growing but most professionals kept a low profile. These events could not be explained by what they had been taught at medical school. This was particularly true with regard to nutrition. Clients that should be suffering from malnutrition, according to conventional nutritional theory, were not only thriving but experiencing improved health in the process. Some of these people had been diagnosed with serious health problems, including cancer and heart disease. Many had been told there was nothing to be done.

Macrobiotic Principles

For the growing macrobiotic community, this presented a serious challenge. The first generation of macrobiotic health counsellors were food activists, not doctors. Macrobiotics was not "medicine" but a simple set of ecological principles that were at the base of the revolution in nutritional reform. The principles were very simple.

The body has a native wisdom. A healthy body knows how to combat most diseases. In the modern world, our systems suffer under a high degree of nutritional, kinetic, and emotional stress. To stimulate the natural healing response, we must provide basic nourishment, healthy activity, and stress reduction.

The simple truth behind most of the macrobiotic approach to healing was based on a few simple principles:

- The natural healing mechanisms of the body are suppressed if the body is constantly struggling to maintain its own bio/chemical balance.

- Nutrition is the single most important factor in creating biological stress or promoting efficiency.

- Much of the modern diet is directly responsible for the decline in personal and public health.

- A top nutritional priority in healing is the elimination of those factors that are most stressful to the system. These include highly processed foods with chemical additives, simple sugars and refined flour products, trans fats, and meat, dairy, and eggs.

- To stimulate the body's healing mechanisms, a diverse diet of whole grains, beans, both cooked and uncooked vegetables, fermented foods (probiotics), nuts, seeds, and fruits need to be eaten daily for a substantial period of time. Even though nutrition works quickly, it often takes time for individuals to adapt and enjoy a new way of eating.

- Eating a seasonal diet based on organically grown foods that have been well prepared is best. Macrobiotic cooking is a simple and effective way to produce meals that are tasty and maximize digestion.

The body has evolved a number of strategies as protection from pathogens. Our lungs, intestines, and urinary tract all work to eject pathogens from the body.

Body's Protective Measures

We secrete peptides and enzymes to protect our skin and respiratory tract, and our stomach produces the chemical defenses of gastric acid and proteases. These protective measures are in concert with the activities of our commensal intestinal flora. These "friendly" microorganisms compete with pathogenic bacteria, and they can alter our gut environment, reducing the growth of pathogens and inflammation.

Inflammation is our body's attempt to remove harmful factors—such as damaged cells, irritants, or pathogens—so that healing can begin. Most of us have experienced the discomfort and swelling of acute inflammation, but chronic inflammation is of greater concern. Chemicals are released by the cells in an afflicted area, increasing blood flow and the concentration of immune factors. If the immune system is weak the inflammation is allowed progress. If chronic, this process erodes cellular integrity and can serve to cause serious damage with life threatening consequences.

Chronic inflammation has been related to many diseases, including diabetes and heart disease. The link between inflammation and cancer has been known for over a hundred years. Inflammation becomes chronic when, for example, there is persistent low-level irritation. There is a good case to be made that inflammation lies at the root of most of our health problems. Many factors can exacerbate chronic inflammation, including many commonly consumed foods, such as processed meat products, trans fats, refined sugar, alcohol, and many food additives. This relationship is well established and well known. Why aren't patients given a diet that reduces inflammation as part of their therapy?

DIET AND HEALING

When I began health counselling, my first clients had fairly minor problems, such as digestive issues, weight issues, headaches, or general lethargy. I promised only that they should see an improvement within a short time, and I was impressed by the dramatic changes. Most of these clients had experienced their problems for years.

By the 1970s, people with serious health issues were being drawn to the macrobiotic way of eating—a situation which, in turn, drew attention and criticism from the medical establishment. Some of the criticism was well intended and some even accurate, but most was ill-informed and often aggressively territorial. With very little training in nutritional science, we were helping thousands of individuals regain their health, but the medical establishment seemed not to take our success into account.

This is an excerpt from a presentation I made in 1978 at the East West Foundation Cancer Conference. I was director of the Community Health Foundation in London, and I was working full-time developing the health counseling and education program.

At our foundation, which is an information center for preventative medicine, we have had increasing numbers of people coming for advice on health issues. Until about eighteen months ago, I had never encountered a person with cancer who had approached it from the macrobiotic point of view. My first experience was when Mr. Kushi gave a seminar in London for medical people. During his visit, he met two clients who had cancer—one skin cancer and the other with cancer of the spleen. After he made dietary recommendations, he referred them to me if they needed any further advice.

The man with skin cancer had a dramatic result. After three months, all the symptoms of the disease had gone away. There was no evidence of cancer on the skin. His doctor confirmed this after a full medical checkup. He also commented on the fact that he was happy to have lost weight and had an improved mental attitude and increased sexual vitality.

The improvement in the woman with spleen cancer was even more dramatic. After seven months, I visited her home and was amazed with the change in her. When I initially met her, she was so weak she could not walk and was confined to a wheelchair. She had regained her vitality and had returned to work. She had done this without any support. She simply changed her diet. She and others I have counseled on my own have experienced vast improvements, which were verified by medical testing.

Over the years, thousands of men and women who were diagnosed with life-threatening diseases have healed themselves. The remission of cancers, the reversal of heart disease, and the return to health are confirmed by physicians and then classified as "spontaneous remission," previous misdiagnosis, or simply a coincidence. Certainly, most of these events are purely observational; they are anecdotal stories and not scientifically validated. After all, the clients and counselors were not scientists or doctors.

In 1978, Dr. Anthony Sattilaro changed things. Sattilaro was president of the Methodist Hospital in Philadelphia. He had been diagnosed with metastasized prostate cancer that had spread to his ribs, skull, sternum, and spine. His prognosis was very poor. His oncologist told him that he was dying and would have to get his affairs in order. Adding to his despair, his father had recently died of cancer.

Returning from his father's funeral, he picked up two young hitchhikers. He told them that he was returning from his father's burial and that he too had cancer. They casually told him that cancer could be cured with diet and gave him a contact in Philadelphia, my friend Denny Waxman. In spite of his skepticism, the hopelessness of his medical diagnosis, the side effects of his chemotherapy, and his constant pain drove him to see Waxman.

After fifteen months of following the diet, a bone scan and gamma camera confirmed that his lesions had disappeared and his films were negative. All the symptoms of his cancer were gone.

Sattilaro's full story, *Recalled by Life,* written by Tom Monte, was published in 1980; and a short excerpt was published in *Life* magazine. Macrobiotics and cancer were dramatically linked from that time forward. Many other books of macrobiotic healing stories fired the public imagination and gave hope to thousands, notably *Healing Miracles with Macrobiotics* by Professor Jean Kohler; *Macrobiotic Miracle: How A Vermont Family Overcame Cancer* by Virginia Brown, RN; *Eating with Angels: the Neil Scott Story;* and *Recovery* by Elaine Nussbaum. Many of those who were attracted to macrobiotics had been given up on by the medical community. Quite a few were disappointed when they discovered they would have to cook, but the successes were inspiring.

Michio Kushi's macrobiotic dietary suggestions do not seem radical now. He advised that all diets have whole cereal grains as their foundation, include a variety of vegetables (preferably locally grown), whole beans and pulses (edible seeds that grow in pods, for example beans, peas, and lentils), naturally fermented soy condiments (miso, shoyu, and tempeh), nuts and seeds, seasonal fruits, and sea vegetables. He distinguished between therapeutic and health-maintenance diets. Most of the therapeutic diets contained very little or no oil and absolutely no fish. Maintenance diets sometimes included fish. Mammal meats, poultry, eggs, dairy foods, refined sugars, and food additives were all considered harmful.

The face of macrobiotic practice altered. Teachers of simple living were transformed into "cancer healers"—a task that they had not signed up for. As before, the medical profession pointed to the lack of scientific backup. The macrobiotic community consistently invited research, but to no avail.

However, credibility was building. The *Journal of Nutrition* gave an overview of the macrobiotic diet:

The effects of whole grains on cancer prevention are probably not limited to dietary fiber effects but may also involve effects on estrogen metabolism, glucose, and insulin metabolism and oxidative processes. A wide variety of vegetables are also recommended for regular consumption. The evidence that vegetable intake is associated with decreased risk of cancer is large and consistent and was reviewed in the American Institute for Cancer Research and World Cancer Research Fund report. This report noted that increasing consumption of vegetables and fruits from 250 g/d to 400 g/d may be associated with a 23 percent decreased risk of cancer worldwide. It has been suggested that sea vegetables—promoted in macrobiotics and an important part of traditional East Asian cuisine—may decrease risk of breast cancer and endometrial cancer. These associations may be accounted for in part by the antitumor activities of fucoidan, a sulfated polysaccharide found almost exclusively in brown seaweed, and fucoxanthin, the carotenoid responsible for the color of brown seaweed.

In its conclusion, the report underlined the difficulties nutritional healing faces when dealing with criticism of the "unscientific" approach. The problem wasn't that it had been proven to be ineffective. The problem was that it had not been tested. There was little interest in investigating alternative approaches to healing that involved nutrition.

Some members of the scientific community were realizing that a "whole-foods, plant-based" diet could produce dramatic healing. In 1976, Dr. John McDougall noted that diet was responsible for many of his patients' poor health. He uncovered decades of research that showed the destructive effects of a diet based on animal foods and the healing properties of a plant-based diet. He is now a leader in the revolution in nutrition.

At the same time, Dr. Dean Ornish published the first in a long line of medical studies that drew increased attention to the healing potential of lifestyle changes. His simple program introduced a whole-foods and plant-based diet, moderate exercise, meditation and yoga, and cessation of smoking. His (primarily vegetarian) approach to nutrition was embraced largely due to his high profile, both as an author of best-selling books and as a success in the reversal of heart disease.

The list of doctors who have shifted their focus toward nutrition grows yearly but some have been in for the long haul. Physicians such as Dr. Neil Barnard (the founder of the Physicians Committee for Responsible Medicine) and Dr. Michael Klaper (who was mentored by Dr. Mendelsohn) are both prominent voices for a more natural approach to medicine and particularly vegan nutrition.

Throughout the 1980s, the world's top epidemiologist, T. Colin Campbell, was a lead researcher on the China–Cornell–Oxford Project, a large observational study funded by Cornell University, Oxford University, and the Chinese government. This groundbreaking study and Campbell's best-selling book, *The China Study,* served as the tipping point in favor of plant-based nutrition. Campbell complemented the study with laboratory research that illustrated the effect of casein (a protein found in milk) on cancer growth. He demonstrated that casein can literally activate cancer cells and that plant protein seems to deactivate them.

We consistently see that eating a plant-based diet achieves excellent results in dealing with heart disease, diabetes, and cancer. So what are the miracle foods to seek out? They may sound familiar.

The modern food doctors recommend a complete avoidance of meat, eggs, dairy, and fish. All stress the use of a wide variety of plant foods, including whole cereal grains, tubers, beans, vegetables, fruits, nuts, and seeds.

Most of the diets avoid or drastically reduce oil and suggest avoiding refined sugars and reducing salt. If we compare this with the macrobiotic programs being used for healing since the 1950s, we see that the differences are negligible when it comes to food choices. The major stumbling block has been that one set of conclusions are based on reductionist science and the other on an ecological approach—one is *micro,* and the other is *macro.*

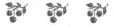

We have made "fighting disease" a straw man to deflect attention from the fact that we are not preventing disease in the first place. The food and pharmaceutical industry together with the implicit cooperation of the medical establishment drag their feet with every call for reform. It has taken a group of outliers—alternative practitioners, social activists, and rebel doctors to slowly turn the tide and work toward a new vision of nutrition. Part of this vision is a deeper understanding of the relationship between what we eat and the natural environment.

Through nutrition, we can find a new understanding of our connection to nature. It reflects our most recent scientific insights with our native intelligence and ancient wisdom. It comes close to answering the second question that I posed to myself many years ago: "Why was this approach to health and diet, based on a system that was thousands of years old, more effective than modern science?" To approach an answer to that question is the aim of the next chapter.

PART TWO

A Natural Perspective

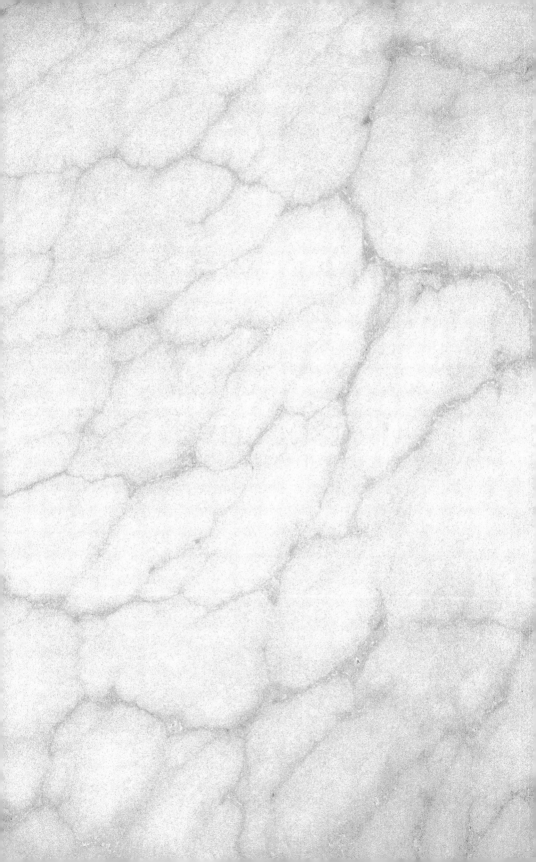

6

*F*ood for Thought

S quirrels don't gather to discuss if they should try a little meat in their diet. Lions don't debate veganism. But we humans chop and change our diets all the time. So how exactly do we make food choices?

It seems that cultural habit, taste, and advertising are the primary motivations that inform our decisions. All are unreliable and derive from emotions or from concepts that we absorb from others. But what if there are biological factors that guide us as to what we eat? We seem to have lost the capacity to detect foods that are toxic. This is an important nutritional issue, especially since the food we eat not only nourishes our body but also our mind.

The degree to which our mental processes are affected by what we eat is a topic of intense scientific study. What we do know is that food + digestion = blood = brain function is a relationship that has long been known. We are only now understanding some of the details but may need to adopt a view taken by some of our ancient ancestors to get a better understanding of how that works.

Americans spend over $107 billion each year on medical treatment for digestive problems. Over 100 million people treat their digestive disorders with over-the-counter remedies. Recent studies show that the second most popular drug in America, Nexium, with annual sales of over $6 billion, and its over-the-counter cousin, Prilosec, are harmful for most people. These drugs, which we use to buffer stomach acid, can cause life-threatening diarrhea, bone fracture in older women, and a variety of other complications. They are inappropriately advised in between 53 percent and 69 percent of cases. So what is the alternative?

Stop eating toxic food! How do you know it's toxic? Well, you know it's toxic because it sets your stomach on fire when you eat it!

Of course, we want food that is tasty, but if it is enjoyable only during the act of eating it and makes us sick after, that's certainly not a good sign. Treating symptoms instead of addressing causes creates disaster. We need to pay attention to our sensitivity to food and give significance to personal experience. We have all the biological features to detect foods that are toxic to us, but we seem to have lost the ability to use them.

HEALTHY CHOICES

Like any animal, we would not have survived without the capacity to detect harmful compounds in what we ate. It is a sign of health when we can discern what actions support our health and which do not. We can look to the past, when the only equipment available was human sensitivity. Those with heightened sensitivity often kept records of their experience, and these insights were formulated into traditional wisdom. The medicine of China, Japan, and India are of special interest since they kept meticulous records for centuries.

Their systems were based on the belief that ordinary people could experience and understand what Rachel Carson termed "cosmic forces." These past civilizations understood nature through the study of plants, animals, and the movement and rhythms of the seasons. They described their understanding in language more poetic than the language of science. The macrobiotic approach to nutrition reflects these ancient insights into the power of food for health and healing.

Macrobiotic Approach

When I was introduced to the macrobiotic way of eating, I was spared confusion because there was little information to distract me from learning about recommended foods and following my personal experience. I sympathize with anyone today trying to make sense of the oceans of nutritional information and conflicting opinion found everywhere they look. The macrobiotic approach can provide a useful compass for anyone attempting to navigate the current nutritional landscape.

Modern macrobiotic dietary practice developed over the past sixty years in America and Europe. It blends the "food doctor" traditions of Japan with Oshawa's interpretation of traditional Chinese medicine along with a modest amount of contemporary nutritional wisdom. The ideas reflect physical, environmental, and social observations and experiences of over five thousand years in the Far East. The modern macrobiotic philosophy about food bears little relationship to Western nutritional science of fifty years ago, but is completely compatible with leading-edge nutritionists that dominate today's thinking.

While the food guidelines associated with macrobiotics are usually the Macrobiotic Dietary Recommendations or the Standard Macrobiotic Diet, it is not a diet in the strict sense. Macrobiotics involves understanding the effects of different foods and making choices according to individual needs. Michio Kushi developed the Standard Diet in the early 1980s assisted by Ed Esko, William Spear, Murray Snyder, and myself. The Standard Diet was originally presented as a pie chart displaying different percentages for various food groups. It was later presented as a food pyramid showing a general model of macrobiotic eating. It was intended as a general template that could be personalized to suit individual needs. You would adjust according to seasons, environment, activity, and state of health.

The model helped people who were seeking to improve their health and those who were dealing with cancer, heart disease, or any other serious illness. And indeed, tens of thousands of people were helped by using variations of the Macrobiotic Standard Diet.

However, while specific dietary patterns may be suggested for specific health issues, using macrobiotic principles with nutrition is not an attempt to therapeutically cure the illness. The macrobiotic approach seeks to assist the body to recover from nutritional stress, which is often the result of the modern diet, and return to biological balance. In the process, the body can generally recover its own self-healing capacity. So people commonly experience a natural recovery of health and, in some cases, a complete remission of serious symptoms. Specific cooking techniques, home remedies, and simple external treatments can speed up this process and may have significant impact.

Since macrobiotics is a wide-ranging philosophy, different interpretations exist. Some interpretations fail to address the environmental, social, or ethical issues that I feel are important in developing a comprehensive approach to nutrition. Some do not reflect the decades of practical experience of myself and many of my associates. For the purposes of this book, I am referring to the dietary standards presented as the Human Ecology Diet, to distinguish it from other points of view.

Macrobiotic practitioners reached our conclusions by a nonscientific route. It turns out that our path was the shortest distance between two points. The macrobiotic view has been proven to be overwhelmingly true. The evidence of contemporary science is that food is now a major contributing cause of many (if not most) noncommunicable diseases and that dietary change can often reverse those diseases.

Today's Science Findings

While science has increasingly acknowledged the dangers of dairy, sugar, processed foods, and meat, the practicalities of creating a healthy diet is still in limbo. Is health really a one-size-fits-all issue? Is the solution simply to avoid the harmful dietary elements and eat what's left?

That quick Google search on "healthy foods to eat" will plunge you deep into a sea of confusion, wild claims, and advertising. There are over 350 million articles with titles such as "10 Healthiest Foods on the Planet," "50 Healthiest Foods for Women," and "Best Superfoods for Weight Loss." Every article claims to be based on science. So what do we choose? Is it goji berries (for the antioxidants), chia seeds (for the magnesium), and kale (for the vitamin K)—or do you just chuck it all in a blender and drink it with some baked salmon (for the omega-3s)? We are still looking at food as a chemical delivery system. As the British philosopher E. F. Schumacher said:

> The extraordinary thing about the modern "life sciences" is that they hardly ever deal with life as such, but devote infinite attention to the study and analysis of the physio-chemical body that is life's carrier. It may well be that modern science has no method for coming to grips with "life as such." If so, let it be frankly admitted; there is no excuse for the pretense that life is nothing but physics and chemistry.

There are over two hundred culinary vegetables in the world and over twice as many fruits, not counting nuts, seeds, and grains. Each has unique nutritional properties; many have exceptional amounts of a particular nutrient. But you do not build a healthy diet by calculations of micronutrients. Science has its limits. Ecological law number 3—"nature knows best." This is a human issue, and to make such a decision, we need to know at least some rules of natural process.

TRADITIONAL MEDICINE

Our ancestors knew about health and nutrition. Indigenous peoples across the world had to learn to survive and flourish in the environment they lived in. Where the environment provided meager resources, the survival strategies were narrow in scope; sometimes the environment was conducive to more elaborate approaches. Many of these traditional practices have been lost. For example, the European witch trials definitely changed the face of indigenous medicine in Europe. With the increasing power of church and science, indigenous medicine was often seen as either superstition, quackery, or the work of evil spirits. The feminist Barbara Ehrenreich wrote:

Women have always been healers. They were the unlicensed doctors and anatomists of Western history. They were abortionists, nurses, and counselors. They were pharmacists, cultivating healing herbs and exchanging the secrets of their uses. They were midwives, travelling from home to home and village to village. For centuries, women were doctors without degrees, barred from books and lectures, learning from each other, and passing on experience from neighbor to neighbor and mother to daughter. They were called "wise women" by the people, witches or charlatans by the authorities.

Acts of cultural suppression have always included the indigenous medical system. Europeans "educated" the Native American population to abandon their language and superstitions in favor of the advanced culture of the European conquerors. But "white medicine" was not much use against the epidemics that Europeans brought with them. Measles, smallpox, typhus, tuberculosis, and cholera were civilized gifts to a population that had never experienced them. Up to 50 percent of some tribes were killed by these diseases, and in Mexico, tens of millions died in epidemics brought about by the conquistadors.

In Africa, too, colonialism halted the progress of indigenous medicine as part of the "civilizing" process. It is true that some indigenous medicine includes trickery, faith, and superstition; but as we have seen, our modern system also has many of the same flaws. Among those systems that have survived the test of time and the erratic upheavals of history are the healing traditions of the Far East, especially those of India, China, and Japan. While not beyond criticism, they have much to offer—particularly in the area of herbal medicine and nutrition.

If science is about the microscopic understanding of food, then these more primitive views are the macroscopic perspective. They deal with the world as perceived by the senses. They are about natural process: how things change in nature without human intervention. These perspectives reflect thousands of years of direct experience and learning. The WHO defines traditional medicine thus:

> Traditional medicine is the sum total of the knowledge, skills, and practices based on the theories, beliefs, and experiences indigenous to different cultures, whether explicable or not, used in the maintenance of health as well as in the prevention, diagnosis, improvement, or treatment of physical and mental illness.

Early hunter-gatherer and agricultural societies developed ecological philosophies based on foods and medicinal plants growing locally. They wanted to understand the food's capacity to sustain health and vitality in humans, and any specific attributes noticeable when it was consumed. These effects would have included, for example, relaxation, increased alertness, improved energy, influences on existing symptoms of illness, dramatic changes in physical function, or useful psychoactive properties.

Over five thousand years ago, the Chinese recognized that diet was key to general health and healing. Diet therapy became one of the four major branches of medicine (along with internal medicine, external medicine, and veterinarian remedies). Recipes still exist for special broths, soups, and herbal drinks from the period. I love this reference to Yi Yin, a famous physician of the period:

Yi Yin, a minister from the founding of the Shang dynasty (1766 to 1722 BC) who had been elevated from a slave to a government official, is noted as also being a talented chef who was skilled at using herbs to create boiled medicinal compounds for curing disease. Historical records note that he wrote a book titled *Yi Yin's Soup Classic*.

One of the earliest physicians in history turns out to have been a cook!

These ancient philosophies were built not by attempting to control nature but, rather, by learning how to best adapt to it. Sometimes these observations evolved into ill-advised or ineffective spiritual traditions, superstitions, and cultural rationalizations. But not always.

The Taoist philosophers (whose observations about nature formed the basis of Yi Yin's approach to medicine) believed that study of the natural process leads to an altered experience of life—an experience that combines instinct, intuition, and our distinctive human intellect. Maximizing personal health was an essential part of achieving this experience. This comprehensive approach to health helps us realize our full potential, nourishes both the body and the mind, and increases our sensitivities to the processes of life around and within us. In the modern age that sensitivity needs to extend out into the built culture of the day and the cultural influences that shape our thinking.

To become responsible consumers, we need to engage with issues, such as public education on diet, the adulteration of food, the environmental impact of our food choices, and the consequences for other humans and animals. It comes down to educating ourselves about the food we eat, establishing our priorities, asking questions, and reading labels.

THE BODY MIND CONNECTION

A subtler challenge, though, is to develop sensitivity to what we eat and how it affects us. This requires developing a visceral awareness of food. We can be sure that our primitive ancestors had more discerning sensitivity than we do today. Their ability to see, hear, smell, and taste the world around them was a survival mechanism. Developing refinement is difficult when our habits are driven not only by culture and emotion but also by a variety of physical addictions.

What we eat affects how our brain functions. We regard ourselves as "the thinking animal" or "the rational animal." But I tend to agree with philosopher Bertrand Russell, who said:

> Man is a rational animal—so at least I have been told. Throughout a long life, I have looked diligently for evidence in favor of this statement, but so far, I have not had the good fortune to come across it.

The human brain is a masterpiece of creation. Our brains have the most complex cortex. This is the part of the brain where communication, memory, and thinking take place. The high concentration of neurons in the cortex allows humans to process more information than most other animals. Our capacity to "connect the dots" originates in the frontal lobes of the brain and facilitates many "human" qualities, such as self-control, planning, logic, complex language, and abstract thought. Within the brain, we collect information about our environment to which we react or respond. There are cultural influences on action and response, but we must pay attention to the physical and biological influences too.

The brain is nourished by our blood. The basic constituents of our blood are the foods and beverages we consume and the air we breathe. The brain uses up to 20 percent of the body's energy, mostly in keeping all those neurons functioning but also for "housekeeping" functions such as cell repair. It utilizes 25 percent of all the oxygen we breathe. Many of the additional vitamins and minerals essential for good brain function are taken in the form of "precursors" within daily food consumption. Precursors are inorganic (inactive) substances that can be converted into active features, such as vitamins and enzymes.

FOOD FOR THOUGHT

During the great migrations of human populations, there were very few sources of fat, salt, and simple sugars. Calorie-dense foods, especially sugars, were valuable sources of energy. Aside from the immediate pleasurable effects of eating them, sugars could convert to fat in the body. According to Harvard University evolutionary biologist Daniel Lieberman:

Apart from honey, most of the foods our hunter-gatherer ancestors ate were no sweeter than a carrot. The invention of farming made starchy foods more abundant, but it wasn't until very recently that technology made pure sugar bountiful.

Salt, too, is essential to good health, and it was much prized by our ancestors. Our body has some of the same responses to salt as it does to sugar. We have evolved in such a way that when we experience either taste, we think we need more. Armed with the knowledge of our susceptibility to salt, fat, and sugar gorging, the chemists of the modern food industry have run riot. Our primitive survival mechanism has been turned against us. We know we don't need this caloric and salt overload, but we find ourselves in the grip of multiple food addictions and urges.

Food Addictions

Steven A. Witherly's report "Why Humans Like Junk Food" is a great introduction to the secrets of the food industry. Food scientists know exactly how to influence the way we respond to the foods they create. Terms like "dynamic contrast," "salivary response," "rapid food meltdown," and "vanishing caloric density" rule their vocabulary. Each term refers to a "mouth feel," and mouth feels can be used to disguise "non-food." The dynamic contrast of biting into a candy that is hard on the outside and soft on the inside is wonderful—unless that pleasing contrast disguises enough sugar to rot the horn off a rhino.

In an interview with investigative reporter Michael Moss, Witherly spoke admiringly of the Cheetos design:

Cheetos is one of the most marvelously constructed foods on the planet in terms of pure pleasure. It's called vanishing caloric density. If something melts down quickly, your brain thinks that there's no calories in it . . . you can just keep eating it forever.

That is almost exactly what we do—we just keep eating them forever. As our survival mechanism shifts into high gear, the hormone dopamine is released in the brain, triggering the reward system, which prompts us to eat more. Food chemists use "super-stimuli" to produce a deluge of dopamine that leads to hazardous behavior. Using MRI technology, researchers have shown that the same neurobiological pathways involved in drug abuse also regulate food consumption. Regular consumption of junk foods leads to addictive patterns and produces withdrawal symptoms when they are stopped. Food scientists do not like the term "addictive." They prefer "crave-ability" or "allure." Who doesn't want a little allure in their life?

We all want to feel good, and we all want to enjoy our food, but we pay a rather large price. We know that the calorie-dense foods that drive the fast-food industry cause, or greatly contribute to, our most common killer diseases. These foods are designed to be addictive. This is not about enhancing behavior; this is about creating behavior. So, do we want our brains hijacked in service of big industry?

One of the biggest-selling drugs on the market is Viagra, which is used for male sexual dysfunction. One of its selling points is that it does not stimulate sexual arousal; it only affects erectile ability. But what if it made you want sex, whether or not you were able, or whether or not you were near a willing partner? Just imagine the chaos that would ensue. Addictive food makes you want that Snickers bar—even if it makes you sick, even if it makes you fat, even if you need to drive to a store to buy it, and even if you know you shouldn't eat it.

Dopamine gives us a sensation of pleasure. The brain likes pleasure, but if the stimulus is too extreme, some dopamine receptors shut down. With fewer receptors, the brain needs more stimuli to experience the same reward. This "increased tolerance" is exactly what the food manufacturer wants you to experience, because it makes you want more! Multiple animal studies show that junk foods become physically addictive in exactly the way that drugs do. The modern diet is closer to self-medication than eating. We have freedom as to what we eat. We just need simple strategies to change our food habits.

Initially, a food addiction is easily satisfied. At first, a small portion of French-fries satisfies you; but with time, it takes an extra-large portion with a few more from a friend's plate to get the "reward." Even when we have had our fill, we might sprinkle a little salt on them so we are attracted to eat more. This is the problem with the "eat in moderation" mantra so often chanted by nutritional apologists for the modern diet. It does not foster moderation; rather, it enables bad habits. That's why the "slow withdrawal" doesn't work either.

Both instinct and intuition are important to any animal, including humans. Any animal can be trained to act against its own nature. Would horses, left to their own devices, run in circles at full sprint and jump over dangerous fences just for fun? Would dogs sit up and shake hands if they were not rewarded or otherwise cajoled? We, too, operate according to nature's rules and can be sidetracked and retrained. We sit up and salivate just like Pavlov's dogs when we see the logo of our favorite food.

A principle of macrobiotic nutrition is that we can become more conscious of the ways that food affects us. Deepened sensitivity—as tens of thousands who have changed to plant-based ways of eating can testify—assists greatly in making the right food choices and dissolving unhealthy eating addictions. The discomforts, if any, are usually emotional and not physical. Go for a few months without any refined sugars and see what a Twinkie tastes like.

The Power of Food

Food is anything we consume, either solid or liquid. All foods affect our brain functions, but when we are locked into an old way of eating, we don't notice. We may be well aware of certain immediate responses to coffee or alcohol for instance. This is because the effects are more dramatic and quicker. But what about everyday substances we eat and become part of our usual chemical profile? People say they yearn for the taste of beer, wine, or whisky; but what if the taste were the same and the brain response different?

I have given several talks to people addicted to drugs, and they have no problem understanding that changes in blood chemistry produce changes in the way we experience the world. Eating a healthy diet involves establishing a "new normal." It is creating a state of physical well-being that increases sensitivity and a deeper experience of how our habits affect us.

Shortly after my introduction to macrobiotics, I had my first insight into how powerfully food affects perception. I decided to try the ten-day rice diet from Oshawa's little book. I went on a week-long camping trip into the mountains around the Little Sur River on the California coast, taking with me only a few pounds of brown rice, a cooking pot, a small bag of tea, and several books. I had been attempting to follow macrobiotic principles for several months but was not very disciplined. For me, avoiding meat and dairy was easy, but sugar posed a problem. It seemed to me that being alone in the woods, beyond temptation, would be a perfect situation to test the power of dietary simplicity.

I spent the better part of the day hiking into the forest. I set up camp beside a stream and cooked up my first pot of rice. It tasted unusually good, but then that's always been my experience in the mountains. Each day I hiked, sat by the river, meditated, chewed rice, and read. The mountains had never looked, smelled, or felt better—even the night it rained. In all my years of camping out and being alone in nature, I had never felt so close to the wilderness that surrounded me. I was eating rice sprinkled with sesame seeds and drinking tea. It turned out that I had more than a ten-day supply of rice, so I continued on to day twelve. I felt wonderful.

When my food ran out, I hiked back to the coast and drove back to San Francisco. There, I felt like an alien from another planet. My perception of my surroundings was greatly altered. My heightened state of sensory awareness was unlike anything I had previously experienced. I did not identify these perceptions as either positive or negative; I simply had a deeper sense of reality.

As I continued my macrobiotic experiment, I noticed other changes. The periodic anxiety of my youth and teens seemed to drift into the background. I felt calmer, happier, and more in control of my life than ever before. As my physical health improved, my emotional life became more harmonious. There was no question for me that my diet and my improved health made me more peaceful and alert.

Over the years, I continue to see the same response in clients and students. Clients usually come to me with physical problems; the changes in their emotional life are an unexpected bonus. They consistently comment on the sense of calmness and clarity that accompanies their shift in diet. One client summed it up perfectly, she said that all the static had cleared up.

The influence of our health on our behavior is generally ignored, except in cases of gross imbalances in brain chemistry or with drug addiction. It is as if our head and our body are not connected. We dismiss the idea that our foods affect our minds unless we are seduced by the dramatic story of a particular food additive or chemical pollutant. Of course, food is not the only cause of emotional distress or destructive behavior, but what we eat does affect our awareness and our state of being. Our physical health establishes a more firm foundation for our whole life and assists in a movement toward our full potential.

GUT FEELINGS

One of the most fascinating topics to surface in human physiology is the relationship between the microbiome and brain functions. The various parts of the body are intimately connected and in constant communication. A feedback network has been discovered between the gut and the brain that goes far beyond messages about hunger. Those "gut feelings" that we may refer to have a basis. Conditions such as depression, a variety of cognitive disorders, and memory impairment can be a direct response to messages from the gut.

We all know that if we have a cold, a stomach upset, or a headache, we behave differently toward the world around us. That world includes the car that refuses to start or the computer that freezes up with the wheel of death. It also includes people. There is no question that even minor health problems may influence us to become more irritable, short-tempered, or vulnerable. We know that our physiology is promoting a difference in the way we respond. Many people are aware that when they drink too much coffee, they become twitchy and nervous. But what if we accept that state as "the way I am?" When we experience a particular mind/body state for a prolonged period, it becomes normalized.

Our habitual way of acting in the world is our own personal "normal." Rather than accepting a pattern of habits and letting them define us, we can adopt a new perspective to understand the basis of these habits and explore how they may inhibit our growth. If the driving force of a habit is subtle, it may escape us completely. It is in this realm that the relationship between what we eat and how we act is most interesting.

The Blood-Brain Connection

The brain is the organ that is most sensitive to changes in blood chemistry. A complex and little understood phenomenon called the blood-brain barrier protects the brain from dangerous toxicity. While the rest of the capillaries in the body allow soluble chemicals to pass through, the cells that make up the capillaries of the brain are more tightly packed, thus only allowing certain molecules entrance. This protects the brain from most infections but makes it difficult to treat many physiological problems with drugs. The brain doesn't allow the drugs in.

Many compounds found in food have been revealed to have promising benefits to brain function. Research into the blood-brain connection has revealed the direct effects of specific nutrients. Chemical compounds such as *Vitis vinifera, Camellia sinensis, Theobroma cacao,* and *Vaccinium spp* (found in grapes, tea, cocoa, and blueberries) each improve memory, learning, and blood flow to the brain.

This does not mean that eating a healthy diet will produce spiritual enlightenment or a dramatic boost in intelligence. Some vegetarians (or vegans) claim that eating plants makes them less aggressive; but of course, many meat-eaters strive for peace in their lives and are compassionate toward their fellow brothers and sisters. I have also met some aggressive vegans. Essentially, we all benefit by having a greater awareness of the world around us. How we eat has direct effects on our sensitivities and can contribute to helping us make better decisions. It is about living up to our full potential.

Precursor Loading

A long-term, healthy, plant-based diet supplies what I referred to earlier as "precursor loading." They are foods such as complex carbohydrates, flavonoids (found in a variety of fruits and vegetables) and beans, some minerals (iron and magnesium in particular), and the water-soluble vitamins. Most commonly, they enhance the function of specific transmitter systems in the brain. Flavonoids, in particular, appear to improve cognitive function.

The effect of precursor loading is seen over months and years. It is not a dramatic shift in perception and behavior; it is a healing process. It is expressed as an increased tolerance to stress, greater ability to focus, and better "executive function." Executive function describes the ability to organize and manage ourselves to achieve our personal goals. It means that we move closer to our true capabilities.

The Enteric Nervous System

The enteric nervous system, which is embedded in the lining of the gut, carries messages from the gut to the brain. This link allows messages to pass constantly from the gut to the brain, and from the brain to the gut. The gut response to our food governs much of the traffic on this internal highway. What we put in our mouth goes to our head. A client of mine who had a long history of emotional disorders says that when they eat well, "there is less static." Dr. Jay Pasricha, the director of the Johns Hopkins Center for Neurogastroenterology, explains:

> The enteric nervous system doesn't seem capable of thought as we know it, but it communicates back and forth with our big brain— with profound results. For decades, researchers and doctors thought that anxiety and depression contributed to these problems (severe gastrointestinal problems). But our studies and others show that it may also be the other way around.

In other words, it may be that problems in the intestinal flora are creating emotional problems. If we eat a well-balanced diet, we don't need to be concerned with the niceties of biochemistry. We just need to ensure we get a healthy range of food without creating nutritional stress. If we can dig down into the bedrock of ancient wisdom, we can find some guidance toward a diet that serves all life.

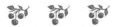

Even when traditional health care is shrouded in esoteric or superstitious beliefs, the origins can be helpful. After all, the beliefs result from centuries of experimentation and observation, and they are firmly focused on survival. Some of them require us to look at our world from a new perspective. We may find the view both informative and rewarding.

7

$\mathcal{A}$ncient Wisdom

U p to this point I have used mostly information from conventional sources. We need to have the concerted attention of scientific view, but it would be a great mistake to ignore the vast store of wisdom that is found in traditional and folk medicine. Thousands of years of experimentation, observation, and recording can be swept aside in the service of more modern mythologies. Often, it is the language that gets in the way. What is interesting is the Macro insights that illuminate a subject as much as the modern Micro way of thinking—that many of the "old ways" and insights are proven to be accurate and effective.

In the introduction to this book, I asked how a system of health that was thousands of years old could cure me and so many others when modern medicine couldn't. As is often the case, insight into the present lies in the past. These traditions most often reflect an attempt to create harmony with the environment. In other words—nature. The laws of nature were the guiding principles. Our modern dilemma is complicated by the simple fact that we live within two environments, the natural primal forces of nature and the built environment created by the hand of man.

LAWS OF NATURE VS THE BUILT ENVIRONMENT

The built environment, the material realities of our life, and the consumer culture demand our constant attention. Under this pressure, we often suspend critical thinking—a dangerous habit in the fields of medicine and nutrition. This is particularly true when faced with the ocean of contradictory "scientific facts" that we are presented with and the social pressures associated with them.

When we step back from modern science's reductionist views, we find many alternative viewpoints. Some of these viewpoints come from the ancient world and offer unique insights into health, human behavior, and our relationship to the environment. Some are spiritual, and some are secular. Some invite us into a deeper appreciation of life, and some may lead to the land of the unicorns. They are not always antagonistic toward science; they simply provide us with another perspective and a different set of concepts.

We know as much about the world we live in as we do about the oceans, which we have explored about 5 percent of. Even science does not know how life began or what the universe is made of. We do not know why hot water freezes faster than cold water, why we create art or why we dream, why we fall in love, or the exact mechanism of the placebo effect. And yet we seem so self-assured in the knowledge that we know the "facts."

Science dominates our understanding of the physical world, and the language of science is powerful. But none of us, not even scientists, live with a physical awareness of the microscopic detail that science is based on. Human beings live in the realm of the senses and the world of feelings. Sensory acuity varies greatly from person to person, and feelings are not easy to analyze; still, they are at the heart of the human experience of life.

There can be little disagreement with the idea that our primitive ancestors were more aware of the natural world than we are. Their lives were dependent on being able to read the patterns of change in the world around them. In his excellent book *Sapiens: A Brief History of Humankind*, Yuval Noah Harari observed:

The average forager had a wider, deeper, and more varied knowledge of her immediate surroundings than most of her modern descendants. Today, most people in industrial societies don't need to know much about the natural world to survive. . . . The human collective knows far more today than did the ancient bands. But at the individual level, ancient foragers were the most knowledgeable and skillful people in history.

The question we should be asking is if that statement about "not needing to know about the natural world to survive" is really true. It is certainly true that we act as if nature is "out there," but that is a dangerous attitude. As long as we can remember our passwords and PIN numbers, show up for work, and pay the rent, we seem to be functional, but the natural world is still around us and within us. And it demands our attention. It is important that we learn to penetrate the static of culture and the built environment. Part of this process is reclaiming our sensitivity to what we eat.

Our Sensory Abilities

We are at our best when our intuition, intellect, instinct, and insight are all in tune and ready for use. This ability can only come when we reclaim our sensitivities. This is simple but not always easy. If our tastes have been hijacked by foods with industrial-strength flavors, we lose the ability to distinguish a simpler way of eating. An apple doesn't stand a chance against a frozen strawberry cheesecake, even when the cheesecake has neither strawberries nor cream in it. What we are losing is "sensory cognition," and that makes us easy targets for sensory manipulation.

One of the purposes of our sensory abilities throughout our evolution is to seek out healthy foods and develop the capacity to detect particularly calorie-dense or nutritious food and avoid compounds that might be harmful or toxic. The perception of bitter taste is thought to have evolved specifically as a protection from toxic and harmful foods.

The implications of this could explain why some people perceive the controversial artificial sweeteners, such as saccharin and aspartame, as bitter. Could it be that these people have a better early-warning system? Without receptors for a particular smell or flavor, animals cannot be motivated to eat or avoid substances with that flavor. Why don't we spit out toxic food we gleefully eat? Part of the answer may lie in the pseudogenes.

Pseudogenes

Pseudogenes have attracted much attention and research regarding our permissive taste buds. Pseudogenes are genes that have either lost their ability to produce the messenger proteins or fail to produce them within a particular kind of cell. They are sometimes referred to as genetic fossils. They are proof of sensitivities that we once had and have now lost. These lost facilities are particularly curious in the case of our capacity to distinguish smell and taste. These two senses are so closely linked that the smell of a food changes the way that the body "tastes" it. Around 60 percent of human olfactory receptor genes are, in fact, pseudogenes, compared with only about 30 percent in other apes and 20 percent in mice and dogs. Your dog may have a better defense system than you do.

If we overindulge we may find ourselves dissatisfied, so we eat more to make up for it. The mind thinks that quantity can offset quality. This corruptible aspect of flavor affects diet, eating habits, self-image—our whole life. Reclaiming our sensitivity requires personal exposure to a simpler way of eating. That is the only way to reclaim our innate ability to govern our appetites and appreciate the diversity of taste and pleasure in simple foods. It may even contribute to our ability to realize a new experience that is not based on outside opinion but on something much more intimate.

LESSONS FROM NATURAL PROCESS

The language of the ancient forms of understanding food is filled with metaphor and poetry. Foods may be described as being wet or dry or cold or hot—even enlivening or relaxing.

Many of these metaphors represent "macro-effects," influences of broader environmental factors than the "micro-effects" of material analysis. The language of macro-effects express the patterns and rhythms of the natural world and also the dynamic forces that unite the observer with the observed. As we will see, food is one of those unifiers. It reflects Einstein's "order lying behind the appearance" and Rachel Carson's "cosmic forces."

Modern physics tells us that all phenomena are composed of an energy that enlivens and connects everything. This reflects Barry Commoner's first rule of ecology: "Everything is connected." This is most deeply experienced through macro-effects. This is the feeling of being "one with" the environment or other people. Many observations in modern physics are consistent with those from ancient cultures. A modern group of observers might attempt to understand natural order by using mathematics and technology. An ancient group might sit quietly and observe the way that water moves in a river or the way that plants and animals interact. Both can come to very similar conclusions and yet express their observations quite differently.

We have seen how our food choices are reflected in society, environment, the economy, and our health. These are examples of the connectedness—the "macro-effects" that we can easily observe. Since we cannot analyse any chemical connection between the environment and the economy or social attitudes and personal health, we need to cultivate different ways of appreciating these connections. It may mean we need to revisit the past to understand the present.

Fritjof Capra was a physicist who wrote the *Tao of Physics*, an attempt to illustrate the connection between the modern and ancient perspectives. He relates this conversation with Werner Heisenberg, one of the fathers of quantum theory and recipient of the Nobel Prize for Physics. They were discussing ancient Taoist ideas as reflected in modern theory.

> I had several discussions with Heisenberg. I lived in England then [circa 1972], and I visited him several times in Munich and showed him the whole manuscript chapter by chapter. [. . .] He said that he was well aware of these parallels. While he was working on quantum theory, he went to India to lecture and [. . .] talked a lot with Tagore about Indian philosophy. Heisenberg told me that these talks had helped him a lot with his work in physics, because they showed him that all these new ideas in quantum physics were, in fact, not all that crazy. He realized there was, in fact, a whole culture that subscribed to very similar ideas. Heisenberg said that this was a great help for him. Niels Bohr had a similar experience when he went to China.

The giants of modern physics—such as Niels Bohr, Heisenberg, Erwin Schrodinger, Bertrand Russell, Robert Oppenheimer, and David Bohm—were all very clear that modern physics was moving through territory previously explored in the ancient world.

For a parallel to the lesson of atomic theory . . . [we must turn] to those kinds of epistemological problems with which already thinkers like the Buddha and Lao Tzu have been confronted, when trying to harmonize our position as spectators and actors in the great drama of existence.

I can hear some of my readers saying "So what? What does this have to do with nutrition?" But physics is the study of nature, both the matter and the energy. Physicists know that the world is not quite what it seems. There are macro-events that animate every aspect of life—including nutrition.

THE TAO OF FOOD

The Taoist philosophers developed a very sophisticated view of the world, focusing on macro-events. If the ancient Taoists lived today, they might be called "deep ecologists." They observed and experienced nature as a living organism of which humankind was a part. Their principal message was that humankind could sense the movement of this primal energy and develop an understanding of its laws. Thousands of years of Chinese philosophy, science, technology, and medicine were based on their insights.

These early physicians focused on individual empowerment and the refinement of consciousness. Attention was directed toward daily routine and developing the will and capacity to change unhelpful habits. The individual was seen to be directly responsible for their own development. Changes might include diet, exercise, meditation, and resistance to social dogma and convention. Modern researchers now agree with the Taoists: the food we eat, the activities we engage in, and the thoughts we think either promote or suppress our true potential for health and happiness.

Psychoneuroimmunology research investigates the effects of emotional and mental states on our physical health. Current research shows a profound relationship between mental attitudes and recovery from disease. The practical uses of this knowledge are often found in ancient practices and live on in techniques, such as visualization, affirmation, and various forms of autogenic training, used in healing.

Epigenetics

This relationship between mental attitudes and recovery from disease—coupled with discoveries about how lifestyle and environment affect DNA cellular functions—opens another window into an ancient understanding of human life. The science of epigenetics is one modern expression of these principles. The idea that a genetic predisposition toward a particular disease is only a tendency and relies on a physical or environmental stimulus to express itself is currently being studied. Nutrition has already proven to be very significant in this process.

Research indicates that some foods seem to stimulate the growth of cancer cells, while others suppress that growth. Professor T .Colin Campbell and his colleagues at Cornell University have demonstrated this "switching on and off" of cancer cells with animal protein. A life choice (in this case, eating meat and dairy) can contribute to the acceleration of a fatal disease. In many cases, this means that by choosing the right foods, disease can be reversed. The renowned physician and Nobel Prize winner Albert Schweitzer said, "The doctor of the future will be oneself." That future is now.

The energy that we receive from air, water, and food comprise the major part of our bioenergetic needs, and it is measurable. Unfortunately, only the quantities are measurable; the qualities are more abstract. Wendell Berry stated,

> The idea that we live in something called "the environment" is utterly preposterous. The world that environs us, that is all around us, is also within us. We are made of it—we eat, drink, and breathe it. It is bone of our bone and flesh of our flesh.

The Pull of Nature

Our responses to the qualities of our environment overlap the edge of physical measurement and our subtler feeling states. We cannot accurately measure *why* the body responds positively to a walk in the woods, but we can measure that it does. We know that being in forests, near streams, or at the seashore makes most people relaxed. This effect is usually put down to the abundance of negative ions; but, surprisingly, showing pictures of nature has a somewhat similar effect.

The pull of nature has profound effects on our mental health. Research shows that exposure to nature and, specifically, proximity to green space causes lower levels of stress and reduced symptoms for depression and anxiety. It also improves cognition for children with attention deficits.

According to the Taoists, either we live within the laws of nature or we break them. Living within the laws of nature is the path to creating a healthy and happy life, while breaking them is the path to sickness. Sometimes the river of life is calm and slow, and sometimes it picks up pace and races down the rapids. Should we resist the stream, or should we consciously move with it? The understanding of these ancient philosophers was that if we closely observe natural law we can align our life in accordance to it. This was their prescription for health—follow the laws of nature.

They continued their studies for hundreds of years, diligently observing, recording, and applying their observations to their own lives. These studies are thousands of years old, yet they could not be more topical.

Micro-effects vs Macro-effects

Western science has focused on the material aspects of cell functioning, tissue groupings, organ systems, and gross anatomy; it is the study of micro-effects. We must consider the nutrient levels of foods; but as we have seen, there is more to nutrition than that. Focusing on specific nutrient values leads to a distorted vision of the usefulness of individual foods.

The Eastern approach attempts to understand the relationships of the parts to the whole. It puts food in context. It is a holistic and ecological reflection of the macro-effects of diet, and it engages with the commensal relationship essential for a wholesome human ecology. It is a way of life that attempts to arrange our life to fit nature, food is one of the keys to this process.

SEASONAL AND REGIONAL EATING

Seasonal cycles, shifts in the weather, and even the move from night into day are not external artifacts. The environment is in constant flux, and we are in flux with it. In the animal kingdom, this shows in cycles of fertility, migration, and many aspects of behavior. These shifts in the environment have influenced human activities, physical and cultural, for millions of years. Our bodies still dance to the rhythm of natural change. Macrobiotics is built around the simple insight that learning to cooperate with natural cycles is condusive to health.

Macrobiotic nutrition advocates regional and seasonal eating to work toward creating balance with where we live, and this reduces food waste and lowers the environmental effect of food transportation. These are both serious issues in the discussion of food choices. The world of international food distribution is topsy-turvy, costly, and wasteful—but it is profitable. Cod, caught off Norway, are filleted in China then shipped back to Norway for sale. Argentine lemons fill supermarket shelves on the Citrus Coast of Spain while local lemons rot on the ground.

International trade agreements mean that fuel for international sea and air freight is not taxed. Cheap slave labor in Africa provides greenhouse salad and vegetables to Europe at far lower costs than local produce. As competition for food becomes more relevant, so does the issue of local and regional food security. Cheap labor like this not only entails shockingly high "food miles" but also undermines local sustainable agriculture. The cheap labor payout, rather than providing security to the host nations, makes them even more dependent on single-export crops. This is corporate colonialism.

According to the consumer group Sustainable America, the average food miles for a watermelon is 1,886. This is because they travel from Mexico. Kiwifruit mileage is 5,015 coming from Chile, and pears from Argentina clock in 5,160 miles. Groups like Sustainable America have advocated labeling to tell consumers how far a product traveled to its final destination.

Perishable fruits and vegetables arrive out of the natural season, and their nutrient levels start to diminish as soon as they are harvested. The industry constantly resists moves to require the seller to provide air miles and environmental footprint information. Knowledge is bad for business.

Fruits and vegetables continue to "breathe" after they are picked. This process (called respiration) breaks down carbohydrates, proteins, and fats, and it leads to loss of food value, flavor, and nutrients. Dry or warm conditions can accelerate the nutrient loss. Vegetables, such as asparagus, broccoli, mushrooms, peas, and sweet corn, have a very high respiration rate and will lose nutrients and flavor more quickly than apples, garlic, or onions—all of which have low respiration rates.

The longer the period of respiration before consumption, the more nutrient loss there will be. Eating a seasonal diet certainly makes economic and environmental sense, but there are other nutritional reasons as to why we might want to eat with the seasons. The body has some secrets we aren't usually aware of.

Seasonal Eating's Effect On Our Health

The environment can profoundly influence changes in human gene expression. Our genes shift quite dramatically with seasonal changes. These shifts affect up to 25 percent of the genetic code that influences our physical behavior, especially the immune system and the inflammatory response. It shows how much our body strives to create a balance with natural process.

Changes in gene expression allow us to adapt better to changes in temperature or other seasonal challenges. We know that seasonal eating helps cut down on wasteful food transport and supports local agriculture, but it could also have a direct effect on our health. If the body adapts to the season, then the foods traditionally eaten at that time of year may well be of assistance in creating harmony with that change. *Homo sapiens* have walked the earth for about two hundred thousand years—that means that ten thousand generations of human life have experienced the changing of the seasons. That cycle is built into us.

Environment and lifestyle influence many complex diseases. Cardiovascular, autoimmune, and infectious diseases and psychiatric illnesses all have seasonal patterns. Scientists are now investigating how our particular environment may be "seeding" our gut biome. It seems that our biological well-being thrives when we adapt to the changes in the seasons. Why should this surprise us? What serves the planet serves us as well.

Seasonal Eating

Seasonal eating has been a hallmark of macrobiotic dietary practice. The foods that are seasonally most plentiful have specific benefits to our body's seasonal needs. They help bring us into harmony with the environment—a harmony our body still craves.

Generally, we find that foods harvested in the autumn are less perishable and can be safely stored during the winter. They hold their nutritional value during the time of year when there is less seasonal growth. They are warming foods; some are known as thermogenic because they initiate a biochemical reaction that produces heat. Some other foods (such as animal source protein) also warm the body, but the effect is more short-lived. The increase in caloric energy from vegetable carbohydrate is not dramatically rapid, but the result lasts longer. Beans, grains, and root vegetables are excellent thermogenic foods for cold weather. Food combinations and cooking can either increase or decrease thermogenic qualities. For centuries, both Western and Eastern cultures have recognized several spices (particularly ginger) and carbohydrate-dense foods as warming, although experiments generally focus on using thermogenic foods in weight loss.

We harvest cereal grains and beans in the autumn and use them more regularly in colder months (although they can be used year-round). Slower-growing root vegetables—such as carrots, onions, parsnips, and sweet potatoes—also release energy slowly. My grandmother served porridge in winter; she said it would warm me all day because "it sticks to your ribs." In hot weather, we naturally choose cooling foods, such as the first greens and early fruits. Foods with higher water content like melons, celery, radishes, cucumber, lettuce, and other salad greens are relaxing and hydrating. They are more valuable in hot weather.

The modern diet constantly undermines the innate intelligence of the body. I was in Helsinki many years ago, and the temperature was below zero. Near my hotel was a supermarket (always a good place to discover what people really eat). Just inside the doors was a huge pyramid of pineapples with a plastic palm tree. A sign on the palm tree said, "The tropics come to Helsinki." Sadly, the tropics were not in Helsinki: no matter how fertile your imagination or how efficient your heating system, nature was in deep winter.

When we eat excessively warming foods (fatty foods, protein) in summer, we crave the extreme: an immediate cooling. Items such as ice cold beverages, frozen desserts, and the like are often used to cool a system that has overheated. Our body suffers the consequences, struggling to adjust to our indiscriminate choices. Foods like ice cream become the norm. Moving back into harmony with nature is a practical process; cooperation with the natural order makes sense. It's how our bodies are made.

A study in Japan discovered significant differences between the vitamin content of summer-harvested and winter-harvested spinach. More sun exposure means more antioxidants in the plant. This makes sense: antioxidants protect the plant from oxidative damage that the sun can cause. Drought and pathogens also change antioxidant levels. In Chinese medicine, the changes in the vegetal growth provide a specific balance for the macro-effects of the season. The season produces the foods that perfectly balance our needs.

Choosing local seasonal foods builds a link between us and the environment, and it integrates us into our world. The two golden rules are to eat as close to home as possible and to try and eat seasonal foods. "Soil and man are not separate." This quote, attributed to Japanese naturalist and philosopher Kaibara Ekken, sums up the macro-effect of eating within the local environment.

MORPHOLOGY, VITALITY, AND DENSITY

In modern science, the study of plant form and structure in biology is called morphology. In many systems of folk medicine, a plant's defining characteristics—such as direction of growth, tissue density, and season of growth—were seen as clues to its nutritional values.

"Ethnobotany," a term first coined by John Harshberger, studies how indigenous people used the plants in their environment. It generally focuses on medicinal herbs used in folk medicine. These traditional plant medicines have contributed hundreds of drugs to the modern pharmacopeia. *Artemisia annua*—used in China for over a thousand years as a treatment for malaria—gave us artemisinin, used in modern malaria treatment. For over two thousand years, the Indian Ayurvedic system has used *Rauvolfia serpentine* to calm violently disturbed patients and as a remedy for high blood pressure. The active ingredient is still used today.

Richard Ford, PhD, from the University of Michigan, said, "Ethnobotany is the study of the direct interrelations between humans and plants." It includes knowing what plants are significant in a culture and how people relate to them. It also examines how people's perception of the plant world guides their actions toward plants.

The world of plants—except as decorative features—is alien to most folks. We want manicured gardens abundant with flowers. We want colorful uniform food plants, and we especially like exotic nonlocal plants. Our "direct interrelations" with plants are virtually nil, and we depend on science to tell us about their nutritional qualities.

There is, however, another kind of science in many indigenous societies; it is an ecological understanding based on thousands of years of observation, study, and experience. Ethnobiology and nutritional anthropology each examines the relationship between food and nutrition from their own vantage point. They consider the evolutionary, social, and cultural aspects of what we eat. As stated in *Ethnobiology* published by Wiley & Sons:

> The extent to which local traditions are considered "science" depends on the definition of science used. The Latin word *scientia* covered cognitive knowledge in general, but certainly focused on knowledge of the wide outside world. The Latin *Historia Naturalis* more specifically covered the nonhuman environment, but could include humans in their relationship with nature. Both terms were brought into English fairly early. Other languages had similar words, not equivalent to modern "science" but comparable to *scientia*.
>
> The Chinese, for instance, had a rich and complex language for talking about knowledge of the "myriad things" and had a thoroughly logical and scientifically analytic tradition, including such things as case-control experiments as early as the second century BC. India and the Middle East had ancient and well-established scientific traditions in constant touch with and greatly inspired by the Greeks. Recently, arguments for viewing traditional Mesoamerican knowledge as science have been adduced very persuasively.

This generous assessment of indigenous culture is not, unfortunately, reflected in the Western practice of medicine and nutrition. This is what Steven Novella—an American neurologist and self-professed "skeptic"—says about traditional Chinese medicine:

> I maintain that there are many good reasons to conclude that any system which derives from everyday experience is likely to be seriously flawed and almost entirely cut off from reality.
>
> It was probably obvious that people need to eat, breathe, and drink in order to stay healthy and alive. But records of pre-scientific thinking about health and disease shows that little else was known.
>
> You cannot, for example, understand how the body works just from biochemistry, or even from studying single cells. You have to understand how tissues, organs, and the whole body works together.

Let's put aside the fact that the Chinese, Greeks, Arabs, and Egyptians had a sophisticated understanding of organs and tissues as well as mathematics before the advent of modern medicine. Are we to understand that since "everyday experience" is likely to be seriously flawed, life is best reflected in a laboratory petri dish? If so, we are left with a study of the body that is detached from its relationship to the environment, the source of its being. That is precisely one of the problems with modern nutritional science; it sees only the micro events that can be discovered in a laboratory.

There has been little research into how macro-effects influence our health. Humans have only recently had the option to eat outside their natural habitat. The modern diet seems a perfect reflection of the built environment. Convenience foods, fast foods, and concentrated foods—characterized by packaging, instant pleasure, extreme flavor, and meager content—could well represent our consumer culture. The modern diet is the food of the urban habitat, reality TV, and social media.

Reflecting on the macro-effects of diet creates a challenge to our consumer mindset. Consideration of the ecological, ethical, and direct health consequences can stimulate and shift our consciousness, especially where diet is concerned. Eating according to natural cycles and macro-effects intimately reconnects our external and internal environments. A healthy internal environment awakens our biological memory and stimulates our health.

We can't examine macro-effects the way we can examine micro-effects. Macro-effects are too broad. They note *general* physical influences and how actions ripple out and impact the larger environment, including society. Macro-effects include our diet's influence on physical experiences, such as heating or cooling, energizing or relaxing, regularity or irregularity of bowel movements, and decreased or increased urination. These macro-effects were central to, and the focus of, the traditional medicine of China.

THE YIN/YANG OF IT

The concept of yin and yang is fundamental to Chinese medicine. The earliest reference is probably in the book *Yi Jing* (Book of Change, 700 BC). The terms *yin* and *yang* were topographic terms indicating the shady side (north) and the sunny side (south) of the same mountain. The sunny side of the mountain represents warmth, brightness, and other characteristics seen as active. The shady side of the mountain represents coldness, darkness, and other characteristics seen as passive. These qualities were metaphors for the flux and flow of energy in nature. The words *yin* and *yang* do not describe "things" but, rather, natural qualities that govern an object or phenomenon at a given time.

Distinctions, such as light and dark, hot and cold, or expansion and contraction, define each other by their opposition. These natural philosophers believed that the interaction of these create all things. We can understand hot because it is part of the hot/cold spectrum; we can identify "up" because it is not "down." For the Taoists, these two partners in the dance of life create the "chi," or energy that produces and animates the diversity of life on the planet. The pulse of this movement is apparent in everything, from the pumping of blood through the heart and the movement of breathing to the movement of sap in the tree and the ebb and flow of the tides. They are the billows that fan life into being.

This energy enlivens the air we breathe, the water we drink, and the food we eat, as well as the emotional and cultural world that surrounds us. For the sages of ancient China, understanding this dance of energy and aligning our actions to its rhythm were essential for living a healthy and creative life. It was their belief that ignorance of this movement brought sickness, unhappiness, and social disruption.

George Ohsawa blended Chinese and Japanese folk medicine with the pragmatic theories of the Japanese food doctors. As early as 1928, Ohsawa taught and wrote about his new interpretation of yin and yang. He classified different features of plants according to certain criteria: many suggested in traditional Chinese classifications and some based on his own insight. Yin and yang describe the two primary movements of energy in nature: expansion and contraction. Energy moving toward a point Ohsawa called yang. Energy moving away from a point, yin. He also identified a number of criteria to classify a food as either yin or yang.

In reflecting on the macro-effects of foods, Oshawa also considered the environment of origin of specific foods. There is a pronounced difference in plant life depending on latitude. Scientists refer to this as the *latitudinal diversity gradient*. The variety of plant and animal life is smaller in the far northern environments and reaches maximum diversity closer to the equator. This diversity is not actually reflected in the abundance of food plants.

Plant life in tropical regions is extremely profuse. In the struggle for life between the diverse elements of vegetation, plants develop survival strategies. Some develop thorns or foul tastes or other chemical deterrents to protect them from being eaten by herbivores. Some of these deterrents are poisons, many of which are powerful and some subtle. A number of the subtler varieties have worked their way into the human food chain.

Oshawa used the nightshade family (common in the tropical regions of Central and South America as well as Africa) as a general example of how neglecting the history of a plant could lead to nutritional problems. This is significant since these plants are known to exacerbate inflammation.

The major advancements in agricultural society happened in the northern hemisphere, which even today boasts the highest concentration of human population. According to radical cartographer Bill Rankin, over 88 percent of the world's population live north of the equator. This concentration of the human population has been consistent since the agricultural revolution.

Using Oshawa's logic, if the greatest number of people have lived in the climates of the northern hemisphere, the foods that are most suited for health are those that naturally grow there. Particularly in those areas with a four-season climate. It is easy to take this thinking to extremes, but a consideration of all plant features can be enlightening.

Plant Features

Plants carry many attributes that reflect the ecological niche and habitat of their origin. These are generally reflected in their structure and form (morphology), thermogenic qualities, and other macro-effects, as well as the micro-effects of their chemical composition. These qualities directly affect our digestion, assimilation, and metabolism, and have shaped our food choices over millions of years. The distinction between root, stem, or stalk and leaf growth is important in understanding Oshawa's classifications.

A specialized group of cells (called statocytes) on the tip of the root instruct the root to burrow down into the darkness of the earth, seeking out water and minerals. This process is "yang," growing downward (which is seen as contractive). It produces a dense form and stable structure. The process is also called gravitropism (for example, the plant is moving and growing in response to gravity). This "tropism," or specific movement, is part of the genetic template of every plant and affects responses to temperature, touch, and season.

The upward thrust of the seedling is seen as "yin." The plant responds to light and atmosphere, expanding and moving up and out in search of air and sunlight—a "phototropic" process.

The divisions in the anatomy of plants are the root, the stem/stalk, the leaf, and the flower (which produces the fruit, seed, or nut). Diversity is very important in healthy eating, so the best diets include a variety of these plant features. Some simple insights into each feature are helpful for food choice and preparation, and for its use with specific health issues.

Roots

The roots (yang) used as food are primary roots. These are from plants where there is a single root, such as carrots, parsnips, turnips, radish,

beets, or rutabaga. The root stores nutrients for future growth and provides stability for the growth above ground. Most of the energy in the
root is stored as carbohydrate. Roots are significant in most traditional
diets. Since they store energy (chi) they are very valuable for providing
lasting strength.

Stems

Some stems, such as cassava and potatoes, develop large storage features called tubers. These are not true roots, although they grow beneath
the ground. They generally do not grow straight down but branch out
horizontally beneath the surface. They are more common in hot, tropical
areas. They are also carbohydrate-dense and are considered more yin
than are the "true" roots. A true root produces one vegetable per stem
(yang); tubers proliferate and spread out laterally (yin). If we compare
the nutrient values of tubers to true roots, we usually see that the tubers
have a higher concentration of calories but a lower density of minerals
and fiber.

Stalk

The upward growth of the stalk and leaf is driven by the search for
sunlight. The stalk is fibrous, to support the leaves, fruits, or nuts. Many
stalks are inedible because of their density, but some (such as celery and
asparagus) are popular foods. Some stalks contain a high concentration
of minerals, which makes them nutritionally valuable. (You will find a
list of edible stalks in Chapter Fourteen.)

Leaf

The leaf creates sugars, and it concentrates proteins and minerals.
Photosynthesis makes leaves generally rich in vitamins. If the root system is the digestive system of the plant, the leaf is the lungs, where
the exchange of gases and moisture takes place. The leaf of the plant
converts sunlight, water, and carbon dioxide into green vegetation, and
it generates oxygen. We know of nearly one thousand species of plants
with edible leaves, which often come from short-lived herbaceous
plants, such as lettuce and spinach.

It is essential to eat leaves as fresh as possible since, because of their
yin qualities, they wilt easily. Wilting is a sign of nutrient loss, especially

of climate-sensitive vitamin C (ascorbic acid). Lettuce, kale, chard, and other leafy greens that are prone to wilting register a higher ascorbic acid reduction after several days of optimal cold storage than does cabbage, which is more resistant to wilting. Small wonder the cabbage was prized in many parts of the world, particularly in Europe. It can be stored through the winter and retain much of its nutrient value.

Differences Between the Plant Parts

Among different plant parts, we can also see distinctions. Density, fluid content, and perishability all come into play. Leafy vegetables with softer edible stalks—such as spinach, lettuce, or bok choy (pak choi)—are more perishable, require less or no cooking, and are more relaxing, cooling, and support healthy excretion (more yin leaves). This is not as true of denser, less perishable, and less watery greens, such as cabbage or kale.

At the other end of the spectrum, roots tend to be less perishable and more hearty. They are denser in structure, dryer, and hold their nutrients well. This means they are often stored after harvest and used in the winter months. Those that mature later in the year and are harvested in autumn and early winter (such as, carrots, onions, turnips, and parsnips) warm the body—perfect for the deep winter months (these are the more yang roots).

Many plants use their fruits as their "seed delivery system." The fleshy part of the fruit often provides nutrients to germinate the seed it contains. In some cases, the fruit is eaten by an animal, who excretes the seed later, thus spreading the range of the plant species. We think of many real fruits as vegetables, including squash, tomatoes, corn kernels, and bean pods. Those foods we think of as fruits are either sweet or sour, and they can be eaten raw when ripe. They are generally classified as yin foods (they are soft, moist, perishable, and grow higher above ground), so they are usually eaten in the season of growth or dried (made more yang) for later consumption.

Cereal grains are both the seed and the fruit (the beginning and the end of the vegetal cycle) and have been the staple food of most cultures since the agricultural revolution. They are excellent in combination with most other vegetable quality foods. Oshawa placed them at the foundation of his dietary theories. They served as the midpoint of his yin/yang classification of other foods.

As Oshawa observed, grains contain the most balanced spectrum of nutrients. They are effectively non-perishable, and they produce the most food per acre. They have, consequently, a special place in many folk traditions and are the most consistently eaten foods on the planet.

In ancient Greece, the grains were the gift of the goddess Demeter, who represented grain, health, and birth. In Japan, the "kami" (or spirit) Inari is associated with agriculture, protecting rice fields, and giving abundant harvests. In the Old Testament, grain is "a most holy part of the food offerings presented to the Lord." In the Americas, the "mother grains" were sacred: quinoa to the Incas, amaranth to the Aztecs, and corn to the Native Americans and Mayans.

Oshawa's students—predominately Michio Kushi—further developed his integration of folk beliefs and contemporary nutrition. The use of grain as a principal food, and the integration of foods from the Asian vegetarian and vegan traditions, are central to the new dietary reform.

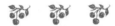

Moving beyond the "Japaneseness" of the original macrobiotic diet requires a more specific focus on the full range of ecological, economic, social, and cultural issues discussed earlier, in order to feed the world in a healthy and sustainable manner. Many of the ideas expressed in the macrobiotic philosophy speak directly to the relationship between society and environment that is essential for a new approach to nutrition.

It has been suggested that a new geological epoch be named the Anthropocene era to reflect human domination of the planet, characterized by the sixth mass extinction of species in Earth history and the continued destruction of the natural world. Species are disappearing a hundred to a thousand times faster than average background rates found in fossil records. Only humans can make the needed changes, and our diet is a major factor in that process.

The changes that are essential require letting go of some of our destructive habits and beliefs. The good news is that when we make these changes the results for our health, society, and the environment are all beneficial. What could be better?

8

$\mathcal{D}$iet and Human Ecology

The biosphere is a delicate and dynamic system of energy and organic and inorganic matter. When we disrupt any part of it, the results ripple out and have far-reaching effects, often seemingly unrelated to their source. Human activity is one of those seemingly unrelated sources for most of the problems in the modern world. War, degenerative disease, the mass extinction of animal species, and the pollution of the oceans all trace back to us.

We have failed miserably to create a way of living that produces a healthy life for ourselves and the world at large. We need a healthy human ecology, a way of living that assures future generations an opportunity to grow and prosper. We need to do it now. We are running out of time.

In 1943, the famed psychologist Abraham Maslow published a paper called *A Theory of Human Motivation*. This groundbreaking work laid the foundations for the next three decades of developmental psychology. Maslow was looking for defining principles of human happiness—for what makes us feel complete. His conclusions were simple yet profound.

In identifying what he called a hierarchy of needs, he established that we must meet our basic physical requirements before achieving other areas of fulfillment and joy. The first level of need includes air, food, water, shelter, warmth, sex, and sleep. When these needs are attained, we seek the second level: safety, protection from the elements, security, order, stability, and freedom from fear. Our desires for love, esteem, self-expression, creativity, and the realization of our full potential rest on the foundation of these first two levels. If they are not met, we risk living with constant anxiety, stress, and ill health. It would be fair to say that those first two levels were talking about health.

When we look at that list of needs for healthy human life it is easy to see that we are painting ourselves into a corner. Those factors of clean water, healthy food, reliable shelter, order and freedom of fear are not available to an increasing percentage of the population. Problems that were once only seen to be common in poor nations now inhabit the streets of the affluent society.

The number of people living in urban areas exceeded 50 percent of the world's population for the first time in 2014. It looks like it will be 70 percent by 2050. The WHO report lists resulting health challenges, such as poor water quality, environmental pollutants, violence and injury, increased non-communicable diseases (cardiovascular diseases, cancers, diabetes, and chronic respiratory diseases), unhealthy diets and physical inactivity, harmful use of alcohol, and increased exposure to disease outbreaks. In an unintended irony, one of the few advantages of urban living is listed as access to better health care (hospitals).

OUR RELATIONSHIP WITH NATURE

When I started studying food and nutrition, I was intrigued by the connection between what I was eating and the environment. I discovered that many of the foods that had questionable or negative effects on health also had an adverse environmental impact. This should not have surprised me.

We do not need new products or even more studies to create a wholesome way of eating. What we need is a new way of looking at the whole issue of food and health. We need a user-friendly, common-sense approach to understanding food that is healthy *and* sustainable for society and the environment. To accomplish this requires us to question everything we have been told about nutrition and review some very basic questions about the role of food in our life and in our culture. Much of the Eastern philosophy that I had read pointed to a particular relationship between the individual and nature.

The word "health" comes from Old English and means "to be complete." Food is certainly an important part of being whole—being connected. To be healthy, we eat food that allows us to operate at our full potential. That potential includes the sensitivity and capacity to adapt to environmental change. Health enables us to nurture the bond between nature and ourselves. Ecology is a central theme of the ancient systems of understanding food.

Ecology is rarely acknowledged when discussing nutrition, and yet it is central to understanding our food choices and how different foods affect us. These effects are both direct and indirect. Rachel Carson, author of the *Silent Spring* and the accepted mother of modern ecology, put it this way.

> If we have been slow to develop the general concepts of ecology and conservation, we have been even more tardy in recognizing the facts of the ecology and conservation of man himself. We may hope that this will be the next major phase in the development of biology. Here and there, awareness is growing that man, far from being the overlord of all creation, is himself part of nature, subject to the same cosmic forces that control all other life. Man's future welfare and probably even his survival depend upon his learning to live in harmony, rather than in combat, with these forces.

This view of our relationship with nature is more crucial now than ever. Carson's vision of an evolution in biological science that unifies human life with the environment has been steadily sidelined. If man is "a part of nature, subject to the same cosmic forces that control all other life," then natural law exists for us as well as for every other creature, plant, and aspect of the planet. If we do not learn to cooperate with the laws of nature, we will harm ourselves. We don't need an environmental degree to understand natural law.

We tend to view the world we live in—and often all other life except, domestic animals—as the "other." Our belief in human supremacy (often referred to as anthropocentric thinking) allows us to place ourselves at the center of the universe. We view our uniqueness as a sign of separation from the rest of life that swirls around us and within us. The belief that we are superior to other life-forms permits us to use the natural world according to our desires and whims. After all, we have "dominion" over all living creatures according to the Christian bible. As we pull away from any physical interaction with nature, we fortify those mythologies that lie at the foundation of our most harmful behaviors.

Types of Organism/Environment Relationships

In ecological studies, there are several kinds of relationships between an organism and its environment. The first thing we need to know about any new creature we discover is how it procreates and what it eats. These are the driving forces of evolution; they dictate physical form, function, and most behavior.

- One class of relationship is called *commensalism,* from the Latin "to eat at the same table." These are relationships where one organism gains benefits and the other is not affected.

- Another type of relationship is *mutualism,* where both organisms benefit.

- In sharp contrast is the *parasitism* relationship, where one organism benefits while the other is harmed.

Creating a commensal relationship with the planet should be a primary goal for humanity. Our well-being is interdependent with the well-being of the planet. It is also the key to a comprehensive vision of human nutrition.

Planet Earth is host to human life. The natural world makes human life possible. Our current relationship with the planet is almost entirely parasitic. The famous British naturalist David Attenborough recently referred to humanity as "a plague on the planet." The chemist and co-creator of the Gaia Theory, James Lovelock, said that humans are "too stupid to prevent climate change." What does this casual disregard for the environment say about us?

We like to imagine that our relationship with nature is a kind of benign mutualism, one where we take from nature in exchange for nature having the pleasure of our company. The conundrum we face is that our whole economy is based on endless consumption; we are eating up the environment. But, as economist E. F. Schumacher said, "Infinite growth of material consumption in a finite world is an impossibility."

Protein provides a good example of a human obsession becoming an environmental problem. Obtaining adequate protein in our diet is easy. A diet with a variety of grains, beans, vegetables, nuts, and seeds provides more than sufficient protein for health and vitality. Asians (who eat less meat than Westerners) have produced concentrated, vegan, protein-rich foods for centuries—such as miso, soy sauce, tempeh, seitan, and tofu. All plants contain protein but old habits die hard.

DO WE NEED FAKE MEAT?

Increasing numbers of people understand that meat is not a good food choice. Some avoid meat for ethical reasons (abuse and killing of animals), some because of environmental impact, and some due to health concerns. Changing to a vegan diet affects social and personal habits. What if you understand all that but like the taste of meat? What if you like the texture of meat? What if you just feel something "meaty" is required. Don't worry; a solution is at hand. Food science is on the way to your door with fake "meaty stuff."

Yes, we can make and sell soy hot dogs, lunch meats, and imitation steaks and pies and burgers. They can taste like beef, chicken, or pork. These products are perhaps culturally fun, but they do not address the issues of good nutrition. Soy is difficult to digest; that is why the people of Asia fermented it. We have to use additives, excessive salt, and extensive processing to get the "meaty" taste that mimics flesh and blood. All because we love to indulge our senses.

Bill Gates has recently backed a company called Beyond Meat. The young entrepreneur who started the company is busy producing all sorts of fake meat in his factory. He outlined his idea in an interview with *Business Insider* magazine.

> Meat is well understood in terms of its core parts, as well as its architecture. Meat is basically five things: amino acids, lipids, and water, plus some trace minerals and trace carbohydrates. These are all things that are abundant in non-animal sources and in plants.

Here we are again in the "food as a chemical delivery system" world. Beyond Meat has manufactured artificial chicken (it tastes just like chicken) and beef in its facilities in Southern California. Ethan Brown, the brains behind the company, has attracted investment from other big shareholders. In addition to Gates and the cofounder of Twitter, the ex-CEO of McDonald's is in the game as an advisor.

Unfortunately many think that fake meat is the best thing since sliced white bread (and we know how that worked out). Fake meat is being marketed as a solution to the "meat problem." But we don't have a meat problem. We have a human problem.

According to Food Research International, manufactured faux meat uses an equal amount of energy to produce as meat products. Bill Gates has taken mistaken paths to environmental concerns, given his enthusiastic support of Monsanto's GMOs as the way to feed the world. The simple fact is that we want to see things change without changing anything. The solution must lie in human ingenuity.

Fake meat is highly processed, manufactured food. It includes canola oil (which is always chemically processed), soy protein isolate (a commercial waste product that populates many vegan and vegetarian foods), and several common additives. It is not a solution to creating a healthy diet. There will be more sophisticated fake meats, some grown in vats like artificial cows, but they still support the mindset that we need meat. More importantly, they give the selection and preparation back to the very same industries that created the problem in the first place.

We have already seen what happens when a good and perhaps ethical idea is bought up by a big corporation. Companies, such as Amazon, Coca-Cola, Pepsi, Campbells, Kellogg's and General Mills, have already bought out several major "natural food brands." In many cases the product formulations are changed, GMO products introduced and general quality of the products has declined. The goal should be consumer control. The only route for that is direct purchase of whole plant foods and the home kitchen.

WHAT IS HEALTH?

I have asked hundreds of students, "What is health?" The most consistent answer is "balance." It's an interesting answer, which speaks directly of the phenomenon of homeostasis. Homeostasis is defined as: "The tendency to maintain, or the maintenance of, normal internal stability in an organism by coordinated responses of the organ systems that compensate for environmental changes." Another accepted usage of the word refers to: "Any analogous maintenance of stability or equilibrium, as within a social group."

Both definitions describe the ability to adapt to change in such a way that we return to a state of maximum efficiency and either biological or social integrity.

Homeostasis involves the relationship between the internal and the external world. This balance between human life and the planet finds its most intimate exchanges in the air we breathe, the water we use, our social interactions, and of course, the food we eat. Our food becomes us. Its digestion can create stress in our bodies, or it can be metabolized with ease. Effective digestion, assimilation, and use are just as important as nutrient values. One of the driving forces in that process is the microbiome of the gut discussed earlier.

Microbes in the Gut Biome

Many microbes found in the human body are not bacteria, but they belong to a very old biological domain of single-celled organisms called archaea. They are thought to be the most ancient of creatures on the planet and are extremely adaptable. They inhabit the most hostile environments: hot springs, salt lakes, oceans, and the human gut. They are usually commensals and contribute to other life-forms without harming them. They make up about 20 percent of the Earth's biomass.

Stanford University microbiologists Erica and Justin Sonnenburg have noted that it is very possible that there are very few Americans who have healthy gut microbiomes. They cite the overuse of antibiotics, sterile living environments, and dramatic changes in our diet as the most possible causes. Central to the dietary issues is the lack of plant fiber in the diet. The biome needs the plant fiber to function. When plant fiber is scarce, the fermentation in the gut is starved of fuel and can't reduce inflammation.

When my wife, Marlene, and I run residential health programs, we feed our students well with the kind of diet described at the end of this book. We notice changes in the participants' health after only about four days. Their moods can improve radically, unhealthy symptoms start to disappear, and skin tones become healthier. I noticed the same phenomenon when serving as the director of natural therapies at the SHA Wellness Clinic in Southern Spain.

These observations make sense. A study published in *Scientific American* noted that with any significant change of diet, the microbe colonies in the gut undergo radical change within three to four days. Lawrence David, assistant professor at Duke University, one of the study's authors, says, "Within days, we saw not just a variation in the abundance of different kinds of bacteria, but in the kinds of genes they were expressing."

An interesting side note is that as part of this study, some participants were fed a plant-based diet and some a diet with cheese and meat. The subjects who ate the animal products saw a significant increase in *Bilophila wadsworthia*, a bacteria known to contribute to colitis and inflammatory bowel disease in mice.

A major function of the gut biome is immunity. In the biome, the immune system can "practice" and develop the resistance to pathogens that may enter the body. Vitamins B and K are created here. It is suspected that even more vitamins are synthesized in the biome that have not been discovered yet. And the biome is essential for the digestion and absorption of nutrients. The metabolism that takes place in the gut helps the body utilize foods that would otherwise not be digested.

Much of what we consume in the modern diet is alien to our evolution. The thousands of new chemicals, the strange new combinations of ingredients, and the eating patterns bear little relationship to our nutritional needs. *Homo sapiens* have existed for about half a million years.

Imagine putting that whole time on a twenty-four-hour clock. At the first movement of the second hand, a human being looked around and wondered what it was all about. For the intervening twenty-four hours, the family of humankind ate a fairly small range of basic nutrients. Then at less than one second before midnight, the system was flooded with over three thousand chemicals it had never encountered before, and with drastic alterations in even the most common nutrients. The result is a uniquely modern problem: nutritional stress.

Challenges of a Toxic Environment

Nutritional stress and air and water pollution are some of the challenges our bodies face as we attempt to adapt to an increasingly toxic environment. But do we want to force our bodies to adapt to such toxicity and then rely on pharmaceuticals to control the resulting damage? If so, then we must expect radical, negative changes in our lives.

As we stray further away from our connection with Rachel Carson's "cosmic forces of nature," we lose track of our identity. Our adaptation to the built environment and to manufactured foods not only undermines our immune system, it dulls our senses and increases our biological degeneration and feelings of disconnection. There is no way to test this premise but it is not too fanciful.

Our cultural environment could not be better designed to create physical and emotional stress. A study by Common Sense Media of over 2,000 children between the ages of 8 to 18 found that those in the 13 to 18 group use over 9 hours of screen media daily. This is more time than they spend sleeping. Those in the 8 to 12 group spent 6 hours a day on media. This two-dimensional world—with no breadth or depth, devoid of a sensory landscape—is the world that the next generation is adapting to. It is not going well. Suicide rates for teens (especially girls) rise yearly. In the USA in 1999, there were 50 girls between the ages of 10 and 14 who took their own lives. By 2014, that number had risen to 150.

Studies have shown that when children are exposed to nature at a young age, their attitudes about the environment and their behavior in nature are reflected in their adult life. Those who have had childhood experiences in the outdoors value the environment more. The problem is that adults spend less time in nature than in previous years. Since 1987, the per capita visits to national parks have declined significantly. This phenomena seems to have begun between 1981 and 1991. Some studies have suggested that it is a result of videophilia (the excessive use of video games). The further we remove our body from nature, the less we care about it. It becomes meaningless.

Nature is our home. Even when it breaks into our busy schedule, it nourishes us. Researchers at the University of Michigan demonstrated that just an hour interacting with nature stimulates creativity and memory performance by 20 percent. This was true even when the weather was cold and unpleasant. A 1984 study showed that patients recovering from surgery recovered quicker when they had a view of trees. Nature calls out to us, but we do not answer. Our social structure is in desperate need of a philosophy that respects our link to nature as something that is essential.

NO FREE LUNCH

Naomi Klein said regarding climate change:

> What the climate needs to avoid collapse is a contraction in humanity's use of resources; what our economic model demands to avoid collapse is unfettered expansion. Only one of these sets of rules can be changed, and it's not the laws of nature.

Klein's words are equally true regarding the crisis we face in feeding the planet. We are literally eating the planet and gorging on its resources, many of which are not renewable. It is a fatal feast.

Laws of Nature

The laws of nature are not abstract; they are concrete and verifiable. Barry Commoner defined these laws of ecology (laws of nature) in his book the *Closing Circle:*

- *Everything is connected to everything else.* Every aspect of the environment is linked; changes in any area affect the totality.

- *Everything must go somewhere.* Nothing gets thrown away; everything has to go somewhere. There is no "outside." Things can be hidden, but they do not disappear.

- *Nature knows best.* Humans have great pride on invented technologies that improve nature; most often the long-term effect of these technologies are detrimental.

- *There is no such thing as a free lunch.* Exploitation of nature will inevitably involve the conversion of resources from useful to useless forms.

If we apply these laws of ecology to nutrition, we discover a number of changes that could create a healthy and sustainable diet for humanity. Other voices, besides food producers and nutritional science, attempt to shout down change. For example, when the UN Panel on Climate

Change suggested that people could skip meat on one day a week to help reduce greenhouse gases, Boris Johnson, then mayor of London, now the foreign minister of the United Kingdom, responded thus:

> No, I am not going to become a gradual vegetarian. In fact, the whole proposition is so irritating that I am almost minded to eat more meat in response. Every weekend, rain or shine, I suggest that we flaunt our defiance of UN dietary recommendations with a series of vast Homeric barbecues. We will call these meat feasts Pachauri Days, in satirical homage to the tofu-chomping UN man who told the human race to go veggie.

The US conservative talk show host Rush Limbaugh also had something to say.

> I know gazillions of beef eaters, and I don't know one of them who has forced his eating choices on anybody else; but I know a bunch of ragtag, stupid vegan vegetarians—holier-than-thou superiorists—who try to force everybody to eat what they eat and to not eat what they don't approve of. Such as this bunch of louts that demanded in Berkeley, California, that Burger King sell veggie burgers—and, of course, Burger King caved.

Famous chef, the late Anthony Bourdain said,

> Vegetarians and their Hezbollah-like splinter faction, the vegans, are a persistent irritant to any chef worth a damn. To me, life without veal stock, pork fat, sausage, organ meat, demi-glace, or even stinky cheese is a life not worth living. Vegetarians are the enemy of everything good and decent in the human spirit, an affront to all I stand for—the pure enjoyment of food. The body, these water-heads imagine, is a temple that should not be polluted by animal protein.

It is difficult to acknowledge the fact that these responses are from adults. (This is not to say that there aren't vegans who haven't grown up yet as well.) Dietary change is an emotional issue and these mini-rants show it. We want to keep eating what we are eating, and we don't want to consider the side effects of our consumption. The idea of significantly reducing or eliminating meat consumption calls forth a telling anger. It is often seen as an assault on manhood, privilege, and domination; it is an insult to comfort and the good life. It is even seen as an unpatriotic affront to our ancestors. The arguments are sentimental; they are not based on either logic or science. They certainly aren't based on the idea of leaving a healthy planet for the next generation.

Cognitive Dissonance

The contradictions we face plunge us into a state of cognitive dissonance. For those unfamiliar with the term, *cognitive dissonance* is the stress generated by holding two contradictory ideas at the same time, or being presented with an idea that conflicts with existing beliefs. To deal with the resulting stress, we avoid any information that rocks the boat, even when it is transparently true.

Most people are taught that cow's milk is essential for good health. In high school, the single piece of nutritional advice I received was from my football coach, who said that if we wanted to be strong, we should drink two quarts of milk daily. That's a lot of milk. So what happens when you are faced with data that shows that milk contributes to osteoporosis, breast cancer, or heart disease?

Even when faced with scientific data and stories of animal suffering, we think of the seemingly healthy milk-drinking people we know, or the happy breakfasts when we splashed milk over our Wheaties. We recall the athletes who have done milk commercials, or we imagine sturdy farmers breaking from the morning chores for a pitcher of healthy milk. Can all those images be bogus? Our resistance derives from a heady mix of advertising, sensory experience, and social habit. We attempt to buffer cognitive dissonance by seeking information that supports our old beliefs or trivializes the new information.

THE THREAT OF CHANGE

The argument that "a little bit won't hurt you" is persuasive. But on the "little bit" route, we end up with a series of half measures that do nothing to change either personal or social behaviors. We want to negotiate with nature, but nature doesn't negotiate. There have been several studies that have shown how quickly and dramatically blood chemistry can change with small alterations in diet. In one study, the blood flow in the forearms of the subjects who were fed a meal high in saturated fat was measured three and six hours after eating. Blood flow into the arms slowed considerably, due to a thickening of the blood, compared to blood flow after a non–saturated fat meal. Other research has shown a similar quick and dangerous change in blood factors that increase blood clotting. These studies show how quickly even small changes in diet can produce negative results.

For example, some people are "Vegan before Six'" or have "Meatless Monday." But if eating animal-sourced foods damages us and the environment and causes the slaughter of billions of animals, we have to questions these tiny gestures. I understand that the motivation of these campaigns may be sincere, but they show a total lack of commitment. If seen in the cold light of day, they are more about making us feel good about a bad idea. They also fortify the idea that animal foods are somehow essential and that we are incapable of change.

The most likely inspiration to improve our own diet comes from seeing the health, vitality, and goodwill of someone with better food habits (and who, with luck, has cooked us a tasty meal). Marlene, my wife, and I generally suggest a three-week experiment of no dairy, meat, fish, eggs, or refined sugars. We give clients recipes and support as needed. Everyone, without fail, has experienced improved health. What they do next is up to them. Small changes may bring modest improvements, but people who go for the complete change experience the best effect and are most likely to continue with a healthier diet.

Healthy eaters tend to get excited when a celebrity eats some tofu, but it is ordinary people who make the difference. Eating well has direct benefits that need to be lived rather than advertised.

Over the past forty years, better-quality foods have become more generally available. Many larger health stores now mimic supermarkets or high-end delicatessens, creating a more familiar shopping experience for some consumers than the funky natural food shops of the 1960s and '70s. An overwhelming number of the products replicate familiar supermarket foods. Many are snack foods. The fundamentals of preparing food from simple ingredients, eating a plant-based diet, and taking control of personal nutrition are still not prioritized.

The natural food revolution has grown at a remarkable pace. A TechSci report on organic food projected the market to have passed $45 billion in 2015. This growth is largely due to increased health consciousness and to increased product availability. Aside from the twenty thousand natural foods stores in the USA, some organic products are now available in three out of four traditional supermarkets. Organic foods now comprise 5 percent of all US food sales, with most growth in young consumers.

But what of the foods themselves? Are they better for us and the planet? Well, not always. In fact, a first-time shopper in a modern natural food shop may get the idea that this is a way of eating for the wealthy. A "generous selection of artisanal cheeses" does nothing to change food habits or educate the consumer. The sun-dried tomatoes from a quaint village in Italy or the specialty beers from Belgian monasteries do nothing to reduce the environmental damage brought about by the transport of nonessential foods. Bucolic pictures of happy cattle grazing in green pastures do not stop the killing of the animals or stimulate any questions about meat consumption. Revolutions are never easy. In his famous, "I have a dream" speech Martin Luther King warned his listeners that it was not the time "to engage in the luxury of cooling off or to take the tranquilizing drug of gradualism." His words regarding civil rights are just as applicable to the present crisis in the environment and our collective food choices. We simply do not have time for half-measures.

RECLAIM YOUR KITCHEN

I was involved in the natural food industry for several years, and I can say that most of the decisions about stocking snack foods and boutique food items are driven by profit, not nutritional, concerns. The only way that the natural food industry will change is through consumer demand. Boutique foods satisfy those who are elitist about good food. The rise of the "foodie" is no gift to genuine nutritional reform. Until we reclaim our kitchens, we are stuck in an upmarket cul-de-sac. Incidentally, reclaiming our kitchens is good for our financial as well as for our physical health—great news since good nutrition cannot be an entitlement of the wealthy. I regularly hear that eating a healthy diet is expensive. My response is "only if you eat animals and don't cook."

Helping Our Kids Eat Healthy

You cannot create change without changing! What kind of immediate changes would help? We always say "Start with the kids." Although if children do not see a serious commitment to healthy eating from adults, they will not take it seriously themselves. Simple nutritional education in schools, including cooking skills, is hugely beneficial. Regulation of school meal programs, in line with sensible guidelines, creates healthier kids. Why doesn't this happen more? Well, for one thing, in America, it would mean stopping junk food companies sponsoring school activities. The uneducated young get their information from advertising.

This may be the first generation of children who live shorter lives than their parents. About 25 percent of children between the ages of 5 to 10 years old have high cholesterol, high blood pressure, and other signs of heart disease. We know where the responsibility lies when the degenerative diseases—traditionally the diseases of the elderly—afflict our children and grandchildren. D. S. Freedman underlines this:

> To be most effective in the long run, public health programs should focus on health promotion as well as disease prevention. For example, by promoting breastfeeding to pregnant women and new mothers and supporting their efforts to breastfeed, public health organizations can help children develop healthy eating habits during infancy. Because appropriate physical activity levels and healthy eating behaviours should be instilled in childhood and maintained throughout life, prevention efforts that target older children and schools are equally important, as are interventions for adults who are inactive or have poor dietary habits even though they have not yet developed chronic diseases.

Unfortunately, changing unhealthy living habits is uncomfortable. It is no different than breaking any addiction. If we blame, instead of showing compassion, it is even more difficult. Luckily, an essential part of our humanity is that we comfort and care for those who are ill and vulnerable. We should harness this aspect of ourselves when encouraging new habits. With the drastic increase of obesity and excessive weight in kids the problem is becoming more visible. You don't need to read a report, you simply have to look around in any mall, anywhere on the planet to see it.

For society to reclaim control of food, we all need to examine our values. We need to better understand our relationship with all life on the planet and the effect of our collective actions. Understanding this relationship will provide the social will to block those industries that damage social and environmental health. The issue of nutrition extends beyond the plate and beyond the confines of nutritional laboratories.

The Nutrition Revolution

The nutrition revolution is sometimes perceived as a liberal attack on the capitalist system rather than a blueprint for a plan of increased health, environmental sustainability, food security, and social justice. These factors and more dovetail easily in nutritional science. The introduction of the "Green New Deal" in congress kicked up a ferocious fuss. Guess what upset people the most? The threat of taking away everyone's hamburgers as topic one. Of course no one really proposed that, but the speakers at a major conservative conference knew how to get the blood boiling. Don't touch my burger!

Nutrition is a very young science. The essentials of a good diet were not discovered until the early 1800s. Vitamins were only seen to be vital in the early 1900s. Research has shown, again and again, that our food is a major (likely *the* major) contributor to the noncommunicable diseases that kill us.

Academic disputes about the influence of specific nutrients continue, but there is general agreement regarding what a good diet includes. Apart from those few highly questionable diets that advocate high animal protein, which I will discuss in Chapter Twelve, the votes are in. A diverse plant-based, additive-free, low-fat diet with little or no refined carbohydrates generally fits the bill.

In November 2015, the Oldways Foundation sponsored a meeting of twenty-one of the world's top nutrition scientists to establish universal principles for better eating. Dr. David Katz, director of the Yale-Griffin Prevention Research Center at Yale University, co-chaired the meeting. Afterward, Katz said, "We disagree about details, but we affirm that experts with very diverse perspectives do have common ground."

However, their "common ground" was pretty ineffective. The experts just basically endorsed the Dietary Guidelines Advisory Committee. While the committee guidelines improve every year, they still reflect undue political influence and industry lobbying.

> The overall body of evidence examined by the 2015 DGAC identifies that a healthy dietary pattern is higher in vegetables, fruits, whole grains, low- or nonfat dairy, seafood, legumes, and nuts; moderate in alcohol (among adults); lower in red and processed meats; and low in sugar-sweetened foods and drinks and refined grains.
>
> Additional strong evidence shows that it is not necessary to eliminate food groups or conform to a single dietary pattern to achieve healthy dietary patterns. Rather, individuals can combine foods in a variety of flexible ways to achieve healthy dietary patterns, and these strategies should be tailored to meet the individual's health needs, dietary preferences, and cultural tradition.

This seems, to me, to reflect a submissive desire to be inclusive. Is our goal a healthy society? If so then let's pursue it. Social habit and economic profit should not stand in the way. There is no "outside" the human body. As the first of Commoner's rules of ecology states: "Everything is connected to everything else." Our patterns of consumption ripple out in the tides of life and wash back to us. Foods that are best for the physical and social environment are naturally best for health. The human body knows that it's winter even if we have central heating. The brain knows it's night even when the lights are on. The ancient memory of the microbiome still knows what to do—if we feed it properly.

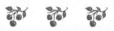

Whether it is Adam and Eve losing paradise in a search for knowledge, Faust trading his soul for earthly pleasure, or Dr. Frankenstein's life being destroyed by the monster he creates, our culture is filled with cautionary tales of man overstepping the laws of nature.

The retooling that is essential for changing course to a more healthy world is not mysterious, as is clearly expressed in the next chapter, it needs to start at the source of the food chain, the soil.

PART THREE

Cause and Effect

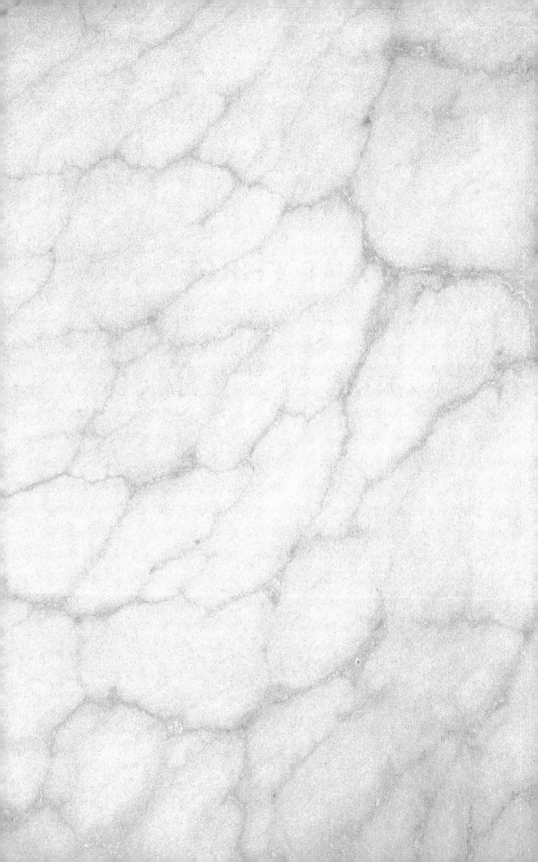

9

The Living Earth

There are several ethical issues that should be included in our redefinition of nutrition. One of these is the environmental impact of our food choices. Food is a result of natural process, a product of our environment. Without living soil and clean water, the food chain becomes polluted. The production of "organic food" is not simply an issue of potential toxicity in the human food supply. It is about life on planet Earth—all life, human and nonhuman alike.

Our bond with the soil is the foundation of food quality. Soil is forgotten in our race to feed cattle and produce ever-increasing volumes of food products. Dead soil is dirt. Dirt is not the life source of a living planet. When we don't take care of the soil, it doesn't take care of us.

Between 1936 and 1940, over 3.5 million people migrated out of the American plains, moving primarily to California. It was the largest human migration in the history of the country. Millions of people were left homeless and destitute. The cause of this tragedy was bad farming. The farmers on the Great Plains did not understand the ecology of the soil in the region.

Plowing deeper using the new technology of mechanized plows, eliminating natural grasses that held moisture, and burning off the fields, farmers managed to kill the soil biome and create loose and fragile soil. Following a drought and high winds, the soil became dust. This dust rose in huge clouds, moving millions of tons of topsoil. Storms blew powdery sand from Kansas to as far north as Boston and New York.

The resulting destruction of small farms meant that large corporations moved in and took over. They used artificial pesticides, fertilizers, and water from deep aquifers, establishing the pattern for the mechanized high-tech operations we see today. The agribusiness replacement is even more destructive than the previous model.

About 60 percent of soil that is washed away through erosion ends up in rivers, streams, and lakes, contaminating them with farm fertilizers and pesticides. This same template has been used all around the world with the same drastic results: dead soil and dead water.

LIVING SOIL

The terrestrial food chain begins with the soil, which supports all life on land. More creatures live within the soil than in any other environment on the planet. It is the single most diverse ecosystem. Bacteria, fungi, insects, worms, and a myriad of life-forms are essential for creating the texture, water retention, availability of nutrients, and general fertility of healthy soil. Healthy plants with high nutrient density are dependent on healthy soil. Any way of eating that undermines healthy, living soil is, ultimately, bad for the planet—and bad for us. Published in the *Atlantic*, the article "Healthy Soil Microbes, Healthy People" emphasized the importance of healthy living soil.

> The single greatest leverage point for a sustainable and healthy future for the seven billion people on the planet is arguably immediately underfoot: the living soil, where we grow our food.

Within the soil, root systems of plants develop intricate relationships with fungi. The fungi function as a communication system. It can even alert plants about the presence of harmful insects or pathogens. Utilizing these relationships increases plant health. When we put intensive nitrogen-based fertilizers (N) on soil, there is a loss in this fundamental relationship. In a report published in Nature.com, the authors report:

> It is estimated that global N fertilizer use will increase threefold by 2050 to meet the growing need for food. The use of chemical fertilizers is often accompanied by inefficiencies that result in pollution and soil degradation. The type and quantity of N fertilizer affects physical, chemical and biochemical properties of soil as well as bacterial and arbuscular mycorrhizal fungal (AMF) communities in the rhizosphere.

These single-celled miracles in the soil recycle nutrients within their ecosystems. A small percentage cause disease (pathogens), but the overwhelming percentage are beneficial and essential. The microbiologist William B. Whitman estimates that the number of bacteria in the world is five million trillion, trillion (a five with thirty zeros after it). They are fundamental to the nutritional density of plants and soil. We are on a mission to wipe them out.

The environments I was most familiar with as a child were the rugged coastlines and beaches of central California and the redwood forests of the Pacific Coastal Range. My father's family were commercial fishermen. Farming, to me, was represented by the small local farm stands dotting the roads in the summer, autumn, and spring—or the flat fields of strawberry, lettuce, and artichokes that grew around Watsonville and in the Salinas Valley. I was in my twenties before I ever met a farmer.

In the mid-1960s, I was working with my friends, promoting what we saw as the natural foods revolution. We sought out those farmers inclined toward natural farming. I was dispatched to take a look at a rice farm in Louisiana. My lack of farming experience was not seen as a drawback. My assignment was to see what kind of people ran the farm and maybe poke around in their barns and see if there were any signs of chemicals. If I liked what I saw, more experienced eyes would follow up.

I was picked up in New Orleans and driven through the bayou country and then given a tour of the family farm. The father impressed me. He loved his corner of the bayou country and was committed to leaving a healthy farm for the next generation.

The family had discovered that they could draw migrating geese onto their land by preventing hunting there (geese are not stupid). They flooded fields and the plentiful food ensured that the birds lingered and fertilized the fields. By adjusting the water level, the farmer could stimulate rice growth and flood out weeds. He talked about life in the fields and irrigation ditches. I had seen the dead water in surrounding farms; but on this property, the waters were alive with frogs, fish, and insect life. He was taking care of the land and was working in concert with it.

One of our main reference guides during that period was a book called *Farmers of Forty Centuries*, written in 1911 by F. H. King (still considered one of the most important texts on sustainable agriculture).

King studied farming practices in the Far East and discovered that the agriculture there was far more productive than in the West. The traditional farmers in the Far East created and maintained living soil that could be productive for thousands of years without the use of chemicals. King's focus on sustainability links directly with what economist E. F. Schumacher would have called permanence. With food production, working toward permanence involves creating a commensal partnership with nature.

FOOD OF OUR ANCESTORS

No one knows for certain when humans started their development of agriculture. Archaeologists, botanists, and ecologists from Bar-llan University, Haifa University, Tel Aviv University, and Harvard University discovered the remains of an ancient camp at Ohalo II on the banks of the Sea of Galilee. This settlement was occupied 23,000 years ago (more than 10,000 years before the usually cited dates for farming of 10,000 BC). The researchers found the remains of huts, cooking fires, scythe blades for cutting grain stalks, grinding stones, and evidence of domesticated plant types, including emmer wheat, barley, pea, lentil, almond, fig, grape, and olive. Similar early planting evidence exists along riverbanks in several parts of the Fertile Crescent and Africa.

Technology now shows us that many (perhaps most) of our ancestors ate significant amounts of plant food. This was certainly true in the temperate regions of the world. Fire was used for cooking food, although it is unclear how frequently; certainly, some meat and tubers would have been cooked. Human life was still governed by seasonal scarcity or plenty.

Our relationship to soil became more sophisticated between 10,000 and 6,000 BC. Agriculture arose in several locations around the world, and it seems to have been a natural progression of man's earlier observations and technologies. Agriculture appeared independently in Mesopotamia, China, South America, Central America, and Eastern North America. There is some evidence that it may have also been present in New Guinea and sub-Saharan Africa.

The agricultural revolution that emerged changed the course of human civilization. Through trial and error, observation and experiment, the great agricultural societies created a new relationship with the environment. Most humans stopped their wandering ways and settled down. This meant that the resources of water and soil required a particular stewardship. For agriculture to succeed, we needed to create a different relationship with nature. We had to take care of it.

Hunter-gatherers faced different challenges compared to agriculturists. More planning and preparation is required when you settle in one place. You have to consider what foods can feed the most people, what foods create the best health, what foods are the most perishable, and, most importantly, how you can create a productive relationship with the soil. You want to work with the soil to produce crops every year, without erosion or lack of fertility. In short, you must create a new consciousness whereby you intentionally cooperate with nature.

When animals or edible plants were overused, the hunter-gatherers moved on. The regular migrations meant that physical possessions were minimal and that smaller tribes were more effective. It required an instinctive relationship with the environment, but not essentially a commensal one. The variations in available animal or plant life, the difficulty in storing food, the periodic relocation to better hunting or foraging locations, or the unintended extinction of animal stock were the driving forces of human life. With agriculture, we put down roots.

As food supplies became more abundant, human populations grew. The more settled way of living—with permanent or semi-permanent structures and the increased use of small numbers of animals in close proximity—brought an unintended problem. More communicable diseases.

Animal diseases, such as measles and smallpox, were easily transferred to the human population. Processing human and animal waste was also an issue. Many of the challenges presented by the Neolithic Revolution are still unresolved and are even more urgent today with increased populations. The settled life requires a high degree of discernment to ensure success without environmental ruin. With billions of people to feed, our relationship with the soil is more crucial than ever.

We are bound to the environment we live in, as is every other creature on the planet. Healthy soil can produce centuries of life-giving food, including all the fruits and vegetables and the grains and beans we need for a healthy life. Productive soil can feed a whole community. Climate (temperature and rainfall), latitude, and altitude determine the organic activity within a specific soil biome. Climate and soil dictate the plants that grow and the animal life that can be supported in any environment. The environment gave us healthy food—as long as we did not overpopulate or destroy the local ecosystem.

SECRETS OF THE SOIL

Humankind soon discovered that areas of rich topsoil in temperate zones were excellent for agriculture. The relationship between the people and the earth began with an understanding of those "cosmic forces" that connect human life and the soil. This relationship expanded into a clearer understanding of the cycles in nature as they related to seasonal changes, planting, care of the soil, and harvesting. We began to understand the difference between soil and dirt.

Soil Microbes

A teaspoon of living topsoil can contain more microorganisms than there are humans on the planet. Healthy soil serves as a digestive system for the environment by breaking down organic material into a form that can be absorbed by root systems. This helps plants to maintain health. Soil microbes not only digest nutrients, they also protect plants against pathogens and other threats. Over millions of years, these microbes have developed a symbiotic relationship with plants. Fungi colonize plant roots and extend out from these roots over a hundredfold. The filaments of the fungi channel nutrients and water back to the plant. The soil biome knows how to manage its own needs. All we have to do to cooperate with the soil is to replace depleted organic matter and get out of the way.

Mycorrhizal Filaments

Recent experiments in the UK showed that mycorrhizal filaments act as a conduit for signaling between plants, strengthening their natural defenses against pests. When attacked by aphids, a broad bean plant transmitted a signal through the mycorrhizal filaments to other bean plants nearby, acting as an early warning system and enabling those plants to begin to produce the defensive chemical that repels aphids and attracts wasps, a natural aphid predator. Another study showed that diseased tomato plants also use the underground network of mycorrhizal filaments to warn healthy tomato plants, which then activate their defenses before being attacked themselves.

Organic vs Conventional Agriculture

No matter what we eat—animal or vegetable—we can trace it back to the soil and the microorganisms that enrich it. When the soil is unproductive, life is damaged. Living soil produces healthy, nutrient-rich food. Studies show that we are experiencing continual soil depletion over time, resulting in poor crop yields. Our current system of agriculture creates declining nutritional value and a sick planet.

The Leopold Center for Sustainable Agriculture's long-running study, comparing organic and conventional agriculture, shows that:

> Farmers interested in transitioning to organic production will be happy to see that, with good management, yields can be the same, with potentially higher returns and better soil quality.

Healthy soil protects against drought by holding water more efficiently, increasing carbon storage (important for buffering climate change), reducing chemical runoff pollution, protecting against soil loss through erosion, reducing soil acidity, and promoting mineral-rich soils. Conventional agriculture creates these problems; healthy soil can redress them.

Promoting healthy soil is as central to the organic food debate as is the effect of toxic sprays. What could be more fundamental in choosing foods for the best nutrition than eating food that is healthy for the planet? The soil's organic life is reflected within us; we are deeply and significantly connected. Wendell Berry wrote:

> The soil is the great connector of lives, the source and destination of all. It is the healer and restorer and resurrector, by which disease passes into health, age into youth, death into life. Without proper care for it, we can have no community, because without proper care for it, we can have no life.

The most recent and far-reaching study on the nutritional value of organically grown food was carried out at Newcastle University in the UK. According to Prof. Carlo Leifert, there are "statistically significant, meaningful" differences, with a range of antioxidants being "substantially higher" (between 19 percent and 69 percent) in organic food. The study, based on an analysis of 343 peer-reviewed studies from around the world, was published by the *British Journal of Nutrition*. It examined differences between organic and conventional fruits, vegetables, and cereals.

The higher antioxidant levels are important. Plants produce many of their antioxidant compounds to fight pest attacks. Antioxidants strengthen plant immune functions. Higher levels of antioxidants in organic crops may result from their lack of artificial, chemical protection, in the same way that children living on farms exhibit fewer allergies, or that the overuse of antibiotics undermines natural resistance. The movement toward organic growing is wise for individuals, society, and the planet.

Organic agriculture can reverse many of the problems of the excessive use of chemicals in farming. Organic farming encourages the use of natural, organic compounds to fertilize soil, maximizing the content of microorganisms that enliven the soil biome. The direct benefits of organically grown food on human health are important, but the long-term environmental benefits may be even greater.

Cover crops, crop rotation, and the avoidance of chemicals promote living soil. It is not unlike creating a healthy gut biome. Organic farming not only saves the soil but enriches it. It increases productivity and produces healthier crops.

KILLING THE SOIL

Agricultural practices increasingly depend on extensive uses of chemical herbicides, fertilizers, and pesticides. These products, along with increasingly intensive production, kill microorganisms in the soil. Many experts question the effectiveness of using chemical fertilizers on a long-term basis. Chemical fertilizers are highly acidic. They reduce the soil biome, increase soil acidity, and hinder plant growth. Changes in the ecology of the soil leads to chemical imbalances in the plants.

The loss of microorganisms in the soil leads to erosion and long-term soil loss.

About 90 percent of US cropland is losing soil to wind and water erosion at thirteen times above the sustainable rate. Soil loss is most severe in some of the richest farming areas; Iowa loses topsoil at thirty times the rate of soil formation. Iowa has lost one-half of its topsoil in only 150 years of farming—soil that took thousands of years to form.

The debate about agriculture and nutrition has become centered on the conflict between organic agriculture and the GMO/agribusiness approach. There are several issues at stake: the direct health effects of chemicals in the food supply, the capacity of different farming methods to feed the world, and the continued viability of soil resources.

The Direct Health Effects of Chemicals in the Food Supply

Although a healthy diet begins with a variety of fruits and vegetables, the pesticides used by conventional growers can have a harmful effect on our health. Since the 1950s, there has been concern that chemical sprays used on fruits and vegetables adulterate the food supply.

DDT

Chemist Paul Müller was awarded a Nobel Prize for the discovery of DDT in the 1930s. DDT was considered completely safe for mammals, including humans. In time, it was seen that while cows that ate fodder treated with DDT seemed healthy, the same was not true of their calves. DDT passed via the milk to the calves, which suffered severe impairment and often died.

DDT illustrates several typical characteristics of pesticides. Pesticides need an adhesive quality that makes them stick to a plant surface. When consumed, many pesticides concentrate in fatty tissues in the body (especially worrying in pregnancy and feeding the young), and many are found in breast milk at a higher concentration than the general exposure of the mother.

A review article in the *Lancet* stated, "Research has shown that exposure to DDT at amounts that would be needed in malaria control might cause preterm birth and early weaning; human data also indicate possible disruption in semen quality, menstruation, gestational length, and duration of lactation." DDT was not banned in America till 1972, over twenty years after its devastating effects were known. Resistance on behalf of industry managed to slow down the use of this deadly poison for decades. As soon as DDT was banned, the Monsanto Corporation introduced its newest poison to the world: Roundup.

Roundup

Roundup is the trade name for glyphosate, and it is used extensively for GMO crops. Research published in August 2010 showed that, at doses much lower than those used in agricultural spraying, Roundup causes malformations in frog and chicken embryos. The malformations found were mostly of the craniofacial and neural crest type, which affect the skull, face, midline, and developing brain and spinal cord.

The research was headed by Professor Andrés Carrasco, lead researcher of the Argentine government research body CONICET. High rates of birth defects emerged in areas of Argentina dedicated to growing genetically modified Roundup Ready (GM RR) soy. This prompted Carrasco's research. Birth defects seen in the children of field workers where GMO (genetically modified organisms) crops were grown were similar to those found in Carrasco's study.

A meta-analysis published in 2014 showed an increased incidence of non-Hodgkin lymphoma from exposure to the glyphosate herbicide. In 2015, the products containing glyphosate were classified as "probably carcinogenic in humans" based on in vitro, animal, and epidemiological studies. Yet the latest agribusiness experiment on unwitting consumers charges ahead. The revolving door between Monsanto and the US government agencies that regulate agriculture and food policies is a much-traveled portal.

GMOs

The director of the National Institute of Food and Agriculture is Roger Beachy, former director of the Monsanto Danforth Center. In 2009, President Obama appointed Michael Taylor as deputy commissioner for the FDA. Taylor was a former lobbyist for, and vice president of, Monsanto, as well as an agriculture trade representative who would push for export of GMOs. *American food policy is bought and paid for.*

Washington-based consumer organization the Environmental Working Group (EWG) found that, in the first six months of 2014 alone, major food and biotechnology companies spent over $63 million fighting GMO labeling. Western lobbyists spent $105 million to fight labeling laws between 2012 and 2014.

The argument against GMOs goes much further than the effect on human health. Monsanto designs GMO crops to provide a constant income stream to the company and to secure control of the world food supply. I know that sounds like a conspiracy theory, but some conspiracies are real. Monsanto crops are patented, and farmers have to purchase seed annually. They can't generate their own. The Monsanto code of business is a supreme example of "green washing." Part of the Monsanto pledge is "Integrity is the foundation for all that we do. Integrity includes honesty, decency, consistency, and courage."

Monsanto is a company at war with nature. The case against GMOs speaks directly to Commoner's fourth rule of ecology: "There is no such thing as a free lunch." The use of GMO seeds is an attempt to control food supplies rather than to feed the world. It leads to lack of seed diversity, narrowing the options for recovery if new strains of plant disease occur.

Pesticides Cause Health Hazards

Powerful herbicides kill organic life in the soil, making increased use of chemical fertilizers essential. This is good for business. In the long term and short term, it is an ecological disaster. To complete the absurdity, powerful herbicides have forced "super weeds" to develop—which, in turn, demand more potent and toxic chemicals to keep them under control. And those chemicals find their way into the human food supply.

The latest revision (in 2009) of the WHO's "Recommended Classification of Pesticides by Hazards" lists about 870 pesticides, all known to present extreme health hazards to human health. These toxins are primarily classified as carcinogenic, as causing birth defects, and as endocrine disruptors or neurotoxins.

Dr. David Bellinger, a professor of neurology at Harvard Medical School, compared intelligence quotients among children whose mothers had been exposed to neurotoxins while pregnant to those who had not.

Bellinger calculates a total loss of 16.9 million IQ points due to exposure to organophosphates, the most common pesticides used in agriculture. The message here should clearly be to avoid foods sprayed with pesticides.

DON'T DRINK THE WATER

Modern agriculture destroys environments largely because it takes so much food to feed animals. The raising of animals for meat or dairy products is, without doubt, the most damaging effect of our modern diet. These animals need massive amounts of precious, scarce food and water. The average water footprint of beef is 15,400 litres per kilo of meat globally. The water is primarily used to grow the feed. So every pound of beef costs the planet 7,000 L (1,800 gal.) of water. I wonder if it would make a difference if everyone who saw a steak was aware of the resources it represents. The World Business Council for Sustainable Development observes:

> Fifty years ago, it was thought that water was an infinite resource. At that time, there was fewer than half the current number of people on the planet. People consumed fewer calories and ate less meat, so less water was needed to produce their food. The volume of water was about a third of what we use today. With a population of over seven billion, the consumption of water-thirsty meat increases competition for this resource. Even more water will be needed to produce food in the future because the Earth's population is forecast to rise to nine billion by 2050. It is estimated that 70 percent of worldwide water is used for irrigation, with 15 percent to 35 percent of irrigation withdrawals being unsustainable.

According to Professor Frank Rijsberman (chairman of the Challenge Program on Water and Food Consortium):

> If present trends continue, the livelihoods of one-third of the world's population will be affected by water scarcity by 2025. We could be facing annual losses equivalent to the entire grain crops of India and the US combined. The crisis has to be addressed comprehensively at all levels, from the way farmers use water to international policy

decisions that affect reforms and investments in water management and infrastructure.

The concept of "virtual water" is used to show a product's impact on water resources worldwide, an estimate of the amount of water "embodied" in the product through its production. Virtual water, when applied to food products, shows the dramatic effect of meat production. Incredibly, beef cattle account for 62.7 percent of water used globally, and dairy cows convert 12.1 percent. Beef uses approximately ten times more water than wheat.

Conventional agriculture not only kills the soil, it infects the waterways and oceans. Chemical runoff pollutes waterways and kills life in lakes and rivers. Eventually, this toxic broth will make its way to the sea, creating "dead zones." These are areas where the nitrites promote eutrophication, causing algal blooms which ultimately lead to depleted oxygen levels and generally poor water quality. There are now over four hundred of these dead zones—where nothing except algae survive—in the oceans of the world.

About 97 percent of the water on the planet is in the oceans; 2.5 percent is fresh water that is frozen, and only 0.05 percent of the world's water is available for drinking. Agriculture is the main pollutant of groundwater, aquifers, lakes, reservoirs, and rivers. Oil, degreasing agents, metals, and toxins from farm equipment often end up in drinking water. So does manure. Waste and ammonia then turn into nitrate that reduces oxygen and kills many aquatic animals.

We need clean water to support healthy agricultural practice and for human consumption, both direct and indirect. A future where clean water is seen only as a product to be marketed has already arrived. When we consider that water is a primary nutrient, our disregard of the quality of municipal water supplies amounts to criminal neglect.

The American Society of Civil Engineers (ASCE) gave US drinking-water infrastructure a D grade in their 2017 report. Among the problems contributing to this poor rating were old pipes that were prone to break, significant leakage, and allowing pathogens to penetrate the system. Often, all these problems were evident in the same system. They cited from between six million and ten million lead service lines in the US leading to lead-contaminated drinking water. Even low levels of lead contamination can lead to damage to the central nervous system in children, learning disabilities, impaired hearing, and difficulty in forming blood cells. In adults, elevated levels contribute to miscarriages and stillbirths, fertility problems, cognitive dysfunction, and elevated blood pressure in healthy adults.

Since its inception in 1970, the Environmental Protection Agency has fought an uphill battle with local and state governments and industry to establish and enforce the Clean Drinking Water Act (SDWA). Every small victory has been offset by increased pollution by industry and social indifference. It is only when the problem becomes intolerable that action is considered. As usual, it is often the poorest communities that suffer the most. Around 95 percent of the population of Puerto Rico are drinking water that is in violation of the SDWA regulations.

In 2015, there were over 12,000 SDWA violations reported from 5,000 community water systems in America. These violations affected over 27 million people (one out of every twelve). These violations included pollution by disinfection byproducts, coliform bacteria, surface and groundwater pathogens, nitrate and nitrite levels exceeding safe exposure, and unsafe lead and copper levels.

If soil is the digestive function of planet Earth, then the oceans, rivers, and streams are the circulatory system. We have blocked the arteries of the Earth and created toxic and anemic blood. As CO_2 increases its concentration in the oceans, it causes higher acidity. This rapid change disrupts sea life, creating decay of coral reefs and dissolving the shells of many species of sea creatures. The impact of this on the future of all life in the oceans would be breaking down the intricate food chain.

FEEDING A HEALTHY WORLD

Water use is only one part of the problem. Great tracts of rain forests are cleared to make way for growing animal feed. Livestock now uses 70 percent of all agricultural land and contributes 18 percent of global greenhouse gas emissions. Our reluctance to consume plant foods (which are superior sources of nutrition) as our main diet is an ecological and economic disaster. The rain forests of the Amazon basin are one of the most important buffers to the rise in greenhouse gas emissions, and they are under direct threat from increased deforestation for growing animal feed and manufacturing biofuels. It is estimated that cattle ranchers and soy farmers alone could destroy 40 percent of the Amazon rain forest by 2050.

By the year 2050, we will need to feed the projected nine billion people who will live on the planet, and our food supply will have to be sustainable—or we will die. Those foods that use soil and water most efficiently need to be the primary focus of a healthy diet. It should be obvious that we will need to stop cutting down forest land and, instead, use the already cleared land to grow food for humans, not animals. If this is not done, there will be no food security.

Foods for a Healthy Diet

Seeds and nuts have been our most important foods, especially over the past ten thousand years of human history. They can be divided into three categories: cereal grains, legumes, and seeds. Among all our foods, cereal grains have the broadest range of nutrients and are the most effective foundation for a healthy diet. They are a valuable source of usable carbohydrate, and they also supply fats, vitamins, minerals, and amino acids.

If cereal grains were fully exploited, they would form the foundation for a healthy human diet for the whole world. They would more than meet human needs for essential amino acids, the famous "building blocks" of protein. According to David Pimentel, professor of ecology at Cornell University College of Agriculture and Life Sciences, the grain grown to feed animals in America alone could feed eight hundred million people.

Whole cereal grains were the foundation of the agricultural revolution and are at the base of most traditional diets. We eat them as porridges, breads, noodles, or simply cooked whole. Some seeds (called pseudo cereals) are classified as either grains or seeds depending on how they are used (for example, buckwheat [kasha], quinoa, sesame seeds, and flaxseeds).

Legumes are beans and pulses. They are a natural complement to grains in most traditional diets. Combined with unrefined cereals, they provide an excellent balance of nutrients. Cereal grains supply our essential carbohydrate, and beans give us more protein and soluble fiber.

Beans are usually prepared by long cooking and even often re-cooking. The use of fermented soybeans, as developed in Asia, has been a particularly useful addition to a healthy, earth-friendly diet.

Cereals and legumes are, without question, the basis of any intelligent nutritional template. They provide the greatest nutritional value with the least environmental impact. For instance, if we take the ratio of water involved in growing alone (without the ancillary processing water footprint referred to above), it takes about 1,800 gal. of water to produce one pound of beef. A pound of rice requires only 343 gal. of water, and a pound of potatoes only 147 gal. A pound of meat, served as a main feature in a meal, will serve two people. A pound of brown rice will provide about six to eight servings (one cup of cooked rice), and the yield of portions with beans is slightly larger. Plants are far more sustainable in terms of water than animal-sourced foods.

Providing for a Growing Population

Healthy food needs healthy soil. So does a healthy environment. Organic agriculture, as I've said, directly benefits human health and society, but the macro-effect is the health of the planet. For true organic sustainability, we must shift from an animal-based to a plant-based food system. We must also implement crop rotation and improved composting methods to replace artificial fertilizers.

Aside from caring for water and soil, we need to care for an increasing population. The number of calories we need, and the amount of protein we can produce per acre, should guide our decisions and be considered as a fundamental nutritional consideration.

Beef produces 1.1 million calories per acre, wheat yields about 4 million calories, and soy 6 million. Rice is very high-yielding at 11 million, and potatoes and corn each deliver about 15 million calories per acre. Despite this, most of the corn grown in America is either fed to cattle, used to make ethanol for use as a gasoline additive, or processed into fructose—probably the worst form of sweetener used by the food industry. Protein values per acre shows the same discrepancy. Soybeans produce 263 pounds of protein per acre, rice 224 pounds, legumes (on average) 94 pounds, while beef production only supplies 15.6 pounds.

The Environmental Impact of Our Diet

In the past, cultures have created environmental chaos and suffered from it. Throughout history, we have created uninhabitable environments. Author Jared Diamond—who won the Pulitzer Prize for his book *Guns, Germs, and Steel*—has written about this in his most recent book, *Collapse*. He focuses on several cultures that have created their own downfall by causing environmental changes. Among them are the Mayans, the Anasazi of the American Southwest, and the Easter Islanders. These were all thriving cultures that destroyed the natural ecosystem to the degree that it could no longer support human life. Our modern world is dependent on the international movement of food. Human society has never collapsed on a global scale, but then we haven't had the physical or chemical technology to make that happen until now.

Over the past ten thousand years, human societies have dramatically changed the environment. The changes were mostly unintended and largely unnoticed since they were so slow that they spanned generations. Now we can clearly see the human impact and have the opportunity to change course if we wish. Human culture has made forests disappear, changed the courses of rivers, altered the atmosphere, and changed the composition of the seas.

Our attitudes to food are a significant part of this process. Many of our foods are extraordinarily destructive to the environment and are not nutritious. People are often attracted to products that promise specific nutritional benefits without regard to their environmental damage. In some cases we are focused on imagined benefits of products with only small or even no real nutritional benefit.

Soy foods, for example, have been popular animal-protein substitutes since the 1970s. This is because of their high protein content, but they have questionable benefits in the way they have been used. By focusing on the protein alone, no attention was paid to the fact that soy, on its own, is not easy to digest. In Asia, soy was almost always fermented or processed in ways that improved digestion. Products— such as miso paste, soy sauce, and tempeh—are processed in a way that increases digestibility and makes the protein more bioavailable. These foods are a valuable addition to the diet but only when processed in a healthy manner.

Another example is palm oil. It has become the go-to butter replacement for vegan products. Manufacturers use it in products like ice cream, margarine, instant noodles, cosmetics, soaps, and of course, cookies. Many products do not list palm oil but simply call it vegetable oil. Recently, in a local natural foods store in Spain, I started to read labels in a long aisle of crackers and cookies. I avoid refined sugars, so the rejects were adding up fast; but what astonished me was that every product included palm oil. There are no exclusive health benefits in using this oil.

Increased demand for palm oil is causing extensive environmental destruction in Southeast Asia. About 90 percent of the palm oil used in the world is being produced in Malaysia and Indonesia. Indonesian plantations alone cover an area the size of the state of Maine, and the area is expanding yearly. The United Nations Environment Program states that "palm oil plantations are currently the leading cause of rain forest destruction in Malaysia and Indonesia." In addition, the United Nations Environment Program found that the Sumatran orangutan, a critically endangered species, is in very high risk of extinction in the wild as a result of logging and plantation development. We are killing these beautiful animals so that we can have cheap cosmetics and cookies. The orangutan population has fallen by about 91 percent during the last few decades.

Official Indonesian data reveal that illegal logging has recently taken place in 37 of 41 surveyed national parks in Indonesia, some also seriously affected by mining and palm oil plantation development. Satellite imagery from 2006 document beyond any doubt that protected areas important for orangutans are being deforested. The use of bribery or armed force by logging companies is commonly reported, and park rangers have insufficient numbers, arms, equipment, and training to cope.

The food industry does not want us thinking about the environmental impact of our diet any more than they want us knowing what's in it. Since the first faceoff in 1977 that I referred to in Chapter Four, the food industry has bought and paid for congressional dietary recommendations that ignore any environmental effect of meat production.

Once again, the DGA guidelines show the power of the big business to effect health:

> There is concern that the advisory committee for the 2015 Dietary Guidelines for Americans is considering issues outside of the nutritional focus of the panel. The advisory committee is showing an interest in incorporating agriculture production practices and environmental factors into their criteria for establishing the next dietary recommendations. The agreement expects the Secretary to ensure that the advisory committee focuses on nutrient and dietary recommendations based upon sound nutrition science. The agreement directs the Secretary to only include nutrition and dietary information, not extraneous factors, in the final 2015 Dietary Guidelines for Americans.

The extraneous factors were, of course, environmental impact. In testimony before the advisory committee for the 2015 Dietary Guidelines, Miriam Nelson, a Tufts University professor, said, "In general, a dietary pattern that is higher in plant-based foods and lower in animal-based foods is more health-promoting and is associated with less environmental impact." The industry wants us to think that environmental concerns are not nutritional. I disagree. Nutrition is the study of how we relate to our environment through our choices of food and how those choices affect both internal and external health.

NUTRITIONAL STANDARDS AND ECOLOGY

The specific directive, as shown above, expresses "concern" that the Dietary Guidelines Advisory Committee "is showing an interest in incorporating agriculture production practices and environmental factors" into their recommendations. Yet in the next revision of the guidelines, it directed the Obama administration to ignore such factors. The food industry will continue to press their cause with vigor—and cash. A myopic view of nutrition, where food is reduced to biological "nutrient delivery systems" suits the food industry to perfection. It distances food from the environment and sees food as an industrial product.

The modern consumer enjoys low prices and apparent choice,

through the scavenging of environmental resources and cheap labor. This wasteful, exploitive system undermines environmental sustainability and food security for us all. As local soil resources diminish, reliance on chemical fertilizers deepens. The resulting expense drives smaller farmers out of business and reduces biodiversity. This is the true *cost* of our present system and is not reflected in the *price* of the food. To discover the true cost of food, the environmental damage needs to be factored in as well as the direct and indirect subsidies and related health costs. The purchasing habits in the wealthier nations are bankrupting the economies and environments of developing nations. The FAO (Food and Agriculture Organization) states:

> Modernization of agriculture has not equally benefited consumers and farmers in the world: rather it has generated winners and losers. . . . The exchange value of food does not take into account the real cost of such systems, so that conspicuous and unreflective consumption is the driver of social and environmental inequality.

The "unreflective consumption" is a result of being uneducated around how food is produced globally. If we are not educated, how can we make sensible decisions? If schools accept sponsorship from fast-food companies and allow junk food to rule the vending machines, how are children to know? We should promote "food literacy" in school and at home.

FOOD KNOWLEDGE

Many children think of food simply as manufactured goods. A recent British study of 1,000 school children aged between 5 and 11 showed some very strange ideas about the origins of their food. Only one out of every three (33 percent) knew that pork comes from pigs . . . And 4 percent thought that pigs were the source of potatoes. Three in ten (28 percent) did not know that carrots grow underground. When I have spoken in some schools, the level of disconnect between what is eaten and where it comes from is seriously distorted. I have heard that food is "yucky" if it was grown in dirt and that it is "made at the store" or "in a factory." (These last statements, sadly, ring true.) And yet the young are interested in the state of the environment. They simply don't connect it with food.

In a recent UK study, it was found that 82 percent of youngsters aged 7 to 14 rated learning about green issues as very important, putting it ahead of science, history, IT, and art. Around 62 percent wanted to learn more about wildlife and nature, and 47 percent want to learn more about where food comes from. Almost all the children were worried about people damaging the planet. An American poll with a sample of 500 preteens showed that 56 percent felt that the world would be irrevocably damaged by the time they grew up. To help, we can educate children to avert and repair environmental damage. The connection between food and the environment is a practical place to start.

When any organism (in this case, man) offends the natural order, there is an account to be settled. This is not a moral directive from an angry god; this is simple cause and effect. When we eat as if life matters, we honor all relationships between animals, soil, plants, the ocean and the air, and ourselves.

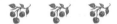

It is difficult to point to the exact moment when we began our steady pull away from knowing about our food. The growth of urban areas and the domination of urban culture happened slowly over several decades. The mass marketing of our food and the erasure of seasonal or regional eating has moved us into a nutritional grey zone. The food in Amsterdam and the food in St. Louis begins to look, smell, and taste the same. It is a dream come true for the food industry.

All this has happened at the expense of the soil we depend on. As industrialized agriculture grows it continues to leave destruction in its wake. Rivers, aquafers, and lakes become bereft of life and simply toxic dumps for the chemical waste of disastrous farming. The damage is not only done to the soil but to those who work on it.

In the next chapter I want to take you to some of the social damage caused by our food habits and the industry that supplies our desires. This is the damage that ripples out from the fact that we seek cheap food, even if it is supplied on the back of human misery.

10

$\mathcal{C}$ollateral Damage

The modern diet is only possible because of the poverty, slavery, and degradation that is suffered by those who produce the food or are trapped in an economic dead-end where only poor-quality food is available to them. We do not often consider where our food comes from, and we think about who did the work to produce it even less.

The idea that every action has an equal and opposite reaction carries a great deal of weight in Western culture. After all, it's one of Isaac Newton's laws of motion. The idea is not limited only to the world of measurable particles but is reflected in many common activities. It is expressed in religions and philosophies from around the world and may be one of the most consistent concepts that unite spiritual thought.

In Buddhist, Christian, and Hindu traditions, Newton's law is expressed in such sayings as "Do unto others as you would have them do unto you" or "You will not be punished for your anger—you will be punished by your anger." Often these concepts are seen as instructions for rewards or punishment in a future life. In the Eastern religions, they are part of karma. "As you sow, so shall you reap." Well, if that is true, there is some very uncomfortable reaping on our horizon.

The modern diet causes huge physical damage. Making dietary changes is challenging, but the fear of disease or the desire to live a healthier life can be powerful motivation. Self-preservation can push us toward healthy eating; however, it barely alters our fundamental attitudes to either food or health. True health encompasses more than measurable physical factors. Health measures mind and spirit as well as bodily functions.

If we make choices out of line with our principles, we find ourselves in a dilemma that undermines our sense of self. But still, we stubbornly refuse to adapt to the unpleasant truth; instead, we tend to freeze or lash out when change is required. But there are consequences—unforeseen and, indeed, unseen—to our refusal to adapt. These unintended consequences often rebound in the suffering of other humans, other species and the damage to the environment. We could call it the "collateral damage" in our war against nature.

Environmental issues are often the solid backup argument for eating organic food or becoming vegan. Why would anyone interested in creating a sustainable planet continue consuming any animal products? Certainly that concern for animals must include the human lives that are sacrificed for our diet. The ethical choice is clear. Creating a comprehensive food ethic requires us to reflect on our concern for all life.

The consumer culture relies on abuses to resources, both material, animal, and human in order to exist. Most of that harm is done out of sight and so easily ignored. In the battle to control world food, the two innocent groups that suffer most are animals and poverty-stricken humans. Their humiliation, suffering, and death are part of the price we pay for our cherished regime: the regime of killing for tasty snacks and exotic delicacies.

FOOD SLAVERY

Let's begin with the humans and let's agree that slavery is despicable and inhumane. Yet, if we agree with that, what do we do about the slaves that produce many of the products we enjoy? Cheap, invisible labor is a driving force of the global economy. This is true of the clothes we wear or the technologies that fascinate us. It also includes our food. Our food is increasingly grown, processed, and shipped by a modern slave population.

Forced Labor

The type of slavery we most clearly understand is forced labor, where a person is considered property and held captive ("owned") in order to labor for their owner. Nowadays, many who are enslaved by forced labor are children—sometimes captured, sometimes sold into slavery by poverty-stricken families. Another type of slavery is bonded labor, where labor is seen as payment for a debt (most often a debt that can never be repaid). Both of these categories of slavery operate in the modern food system.

Agricultural Slavery

Agricultural slavery is as old as human history. The first known agricultural slaves were in Mesopotamia, around 3000 BC. Slave labor drove the agricultural growth in the Fertile Crescent. Slaves built the irrigation systems that made large-scale farming possible. Agricultural slaves were critical to the growth of Western civilization in Greece, Egypt, and Rome. Slavery also drove the economy of America and of much of Europe.

Encomienda

During the Spanish colonial period in the Americas, the economy was based on the exploitation of both land and the indigenous population. The Spanish settlers organized a system called "encomienda," whereby Spaniards were given title to American land and ownership of the villages on that land. In return for Christianizing the local population, the Spanish were allowed to use the land and labor any way they saw fit. This system quickly turned into something very close to outright slavery: indigenous people were paid exceedingly low wages—if anything at all—to perform backbreaking labor on plantations and in mines.

The Spanish professed their God-given duty to convert the local people to Christianity, and more conversions led to ownership of more land and villages. The result was a race for control of people, rather than of land—and not too surprisingly, abuses were normal. Without the use of local labor, the Spanish colonies in the Americas would have failed quickly. The same is true of the European settlement of North America.

Field Workers

Of the 6.5 million immigrants who survived the brutal Atlantic crossing and settled in North America between 1492 and 1776, only 1 million were Europeans. The remaining 5.5 million were African. An average of 80 percent of these enslaved Africans—men, women, and children—were employed as field workers. Only the children under six, the elderly, and the sick escaped daily work. More than half of the enslaved African captives in the Americas were employed on sugar plantations. Sugar became the leading slave-produced commodity in the Americas. Trade in sugar was also a major force in the financial life of England. Agricultural slavery was the foundation of the sugar industry and food crops and also in the growing and harvesting of hemp (for making rope) and of tobacco. The country was built on the work of slaves both for food and raw goods.

Wage Slavery

It is imagined in America that slavery disappeared with Lincoln's Emancipation Proclamation or with the passage of the Thirteenth Amendment to the Constitution in 1865. But immediately after the Thirteenth Amendment was passed, a new form of wage slavery was instituted on a grand scale. This system was based on giving credit to the black or poor white farmer, using the future harvest as collateral. Credit was given at very high interest so that when the harvest was sold and the debt was paid, there was barely enough left to live on through the winter.

The system bound the sharecropper to the bank or merchants extending the loans. Similar wage slavery exists in many parts of the world today. Many would say that most modern farmers with small holdings are enslaved by debt to the system.

The modern slave is well hidden, tucked away in some lonely corner of society disguised as a "low-paid worker" (in reality, a wage slave). We love a bargain, including food. Producing food that is cheap in the market place always means one thing— someone didn't get paid.

THE TOXIC HARVEST

When I was a child, we would roll up the windows in our car as crop dusters swooped over the Central Californian strawberry or lettuce fields spraying pesticides. The fact that the workers were in the field did not slow up the spraying. They could not roll up the windows. There was no protective clothing for the workers, only a bandana tied over the mouth and the shirts buttoned up.

These workers were called *braceros* ("he who works"), and work they certainly did. They worked from sunup till sundown and then disappeared to their small shacks, well out of view of proper society. As long as they disappeared back to Mexico at the end of the season, everyone was happy. Their movement was restricted, they were not paid a living wage, and they were expendable. If they complained or got sick, they could be sent back across the border. They were slaves.

Bracero Program

The Bracero Program was set up in 1942 between Mexico and the USA to bring much-needed peasant workers to American fields. They were needed to replace the poor whites that were either fighting or working in factories essential for the Second World War. They were given contracts that lasted between six weeks and six months, before the workers returned home. The US government protected the rules of recruitment and the rights of the workers until the war ended.

The program was extended under pressure from the agriculture industry that had benefited greatly from the cheap labor. The responsibility for the program passed into the hands of the employers, and the exploitation and abuse of the workers began in earnest.

> Some believe that any guest-worker program, such as the Braceros Program, can be equated with indentured servitude. Linking the legal status of a worker to a binding contract shifts all the power to the side of the employer and will inevitably lead to abuse (Vogel, 2007). Indeed, Lee G. Williams, the US Department of Labor figure in charge of the Bracero Program, described it as a system of "legalized slavery."

The public was effectively oblivious to this exploitation until a series of fatal accidents in the 1950s.

For over a decade, California farmers had transported braceros from field to field in crowded makeshift buses; they were mounted on flatbed trucks with canvas covers. Fourteen men were killed in two fatal bus-and-train collisions in 1953; and in 1958, fourteen men were burned to death when gasoline cans caught fire and the chains binding the vehicle trapped the men inside. These events were seen as tragic but drew little attention outside Central California.

Then on September 17, 1963, one of the converted flatbed "buses" loaded up a cargo of fifty-seven men near the small town of Chualar. They had just finished their ten-hour workday and were going back to the shantytown where they lived. The foreman and driver of the crew and his assistant were checking the time sheets when they drove over an unmarked train track; they did not hear the whistle of an approaching train. The men didn't have a chance. Twenty-three were killed instantly; the death toll eventually reached thirty-one. The conditions of the workers finally received some attention, and the event eventually proved to be a stimulus for the emerging Chicano civil rights movement.

The author Truman E. Moore referred to the braceros as "the slaves we rent." There were several local and federal investigations, a criminal trial for the driver (who was acquitted), and a public funeral attended by public officials. But there was no punishment or blame placed on the growers. Mexican American congressman Henry Gonzalez lobbied for change, but the state government and newspapers rallied behind the growers. A local newspaper condemned critics of the bracero program as uninformed and emotional. The editorial summed up the situation as this:

> We must not let our shock and heartsick feelings spread and endanger a worthwhile farm labor program that has solved the age-old problem of how to get our produce to market in the most feasible way.

The proper definition of *feasible* would be "profitable."

What some politicians in America now see as a Mexican immigration problem grew out of a government policy that was hijacked by agribusiness as a supply of cheap labor. Once the flow of legal workers began, it was easy for impoverished people to cross the border illegally and find work. In the Salinas valley, low-priced salad vegetables were plentiful all year round because Mexican workers were being exploited by California growers. But the problem is not only in California.

THE MODERN SLAVE TRADE

Over 1,200 people have been freed from slave rings in Florida during the past decade. Since 1997, the Justice Department has prosecuted seven slavery cases in Florida, four involving tomato and citrus harvesters. The Coalition of Immokalee Workers has brought the abysmal state of human rights in US agriculture to public light, and it has been successful in pursuing nine cases of abuse against outlaw growers. The workers—mostly indigenous Mexicans and Guatemalans—were forced to work ten- to twelve-hour days, six days per week, for as little as $20 per week. They were under the constant watch of armed guards. Those who attempted to escape were assaulted, pistol-whipped, and even shot.

Guest Workers

In September 2010, staff of guest-worker recruiting giant Global Horizons were charged with operating a forced labor ring active in thirteen states, including Florida. Global Horizons, the CEO, and six others were accused of holding six hundred "guest workers" from Thailand against their will in what prosecutors called "the largest human trafficking case in US history."

Strawberry Workers

In the UK, both Tesco and Sainsbury supermarket chains launched an investigation of suppliers of strawberry workers. To extend the season from six weeks to six months, suppliers of the fruit hire Eastern European workers to work in "poly tunnel" farms. The workers are said to work up to 14 hour days, seven days a week for pennies. They are charged for lodging and meager food and are often in debt when their season ends. The same situation exists for strawberry pickers in Mexico where workers rebelled and closed the roads to draw attention to their abuse.

Palm Oil Production

Today's food slaves are generally out of sight, in other countries. Palm oil plantations in Malaysia continue to draw attention as centers for human trafficking. Forced labor and debt bondage are common. Dunkin Donuts, Girl Scout Cookies, and most of the mass-produced baked products that flood the market use palm oil. *Bloomberg Businessweek* magazine and the Rainforest Action Network stated that Cargill, one of the world's largest food companies, was receiving direct supplies of palm oil produced by contract companies using slaves.

Banana Workers

Americans and Europeans love bananas; they are one of the top five food crops in the world. They are often touted as miracle foods and feature in endless smoothies and diet programs. Many people will tell you they eat them because they are high in potassium; most fruits are. The truth is, we like the taste and mouth feel. We want them at any price.

In July 2010, a Los Angeles judge overturned a previous ruling that had awarded $2.3 million in compensation to six Nicaraguan banana workers. Dole Food Company, the workers' former employer, had authorized the administration of dangerous pesticides (mainly Fumazone) that left the men sterile.

Many of the bananas consumed by the affluent used to come from Nicaragua. It was here that Dole Fruit, Chiquita Bananas, Shell, and Occidental Chemical came under fire in as early as 1986 when the companies were found at fault and the workers were granted compensation. By 2010, the ruling had been reversed by a judge who found that a California court had little interest in punishing a US corporation for actions outside US borders. The industry has now moved on to other countries in Central America and Western Africa. The workers are still employed at the whim of the internationals.

Greenhouses of Almeria

In Spain, the greenhouses of Almeria are peopled by thousands of migrants from North Africa. They produce the peppers, tomatoes, cucumbers, and courgettes that grace the colorful supermarket displays of Northern Europe. The Red Cross has handed out free food to these migrants and described the situation as "inhuman."

Sadly, inhuman conditions infect every aspect of the multinational food chain. Wage-slave banana farmers in Costa Rica are poisoned with toxic herbicides. Women's hands are permanently disfigured by acidic oil film on the nuts in the Indian cashew industry. It is the poor of the world who suffer the real cost of our uninformed food choices. George Orwell stated,

> Under the capitalist system, in order that England may live in comparative comfort, a hundred million Indians must live on the verge of starvation—an evil state of affairs, but you acquiesce in it every time you step into a taxi or eat a plate of strawberries and cream.

MODERN PIRATES AND KILLERS FOR HIRE

The worst kind of modern slavery operates in the Indonesian fishing industry. Cambodian and Burmese men are captured to work on the fishing fleets that scour the Indonesian waters. The Thai government has failed to control these fleets, where men are often chained to the boats and can be sold from ship to ship. The Nestlé Corporation admitted that it was "difficult" to control fish sources due to multiple ports and the fishing vessels operating in international waters. Much of the "fish product" produced through this human misery is used in cat food. Even our pets can have slaves.

Slave Boats

An investigation by the *Guardian* called attention to shrimp boats running out of Thailand. One-third of all shrimp imported into America comes from Thailand. We do love cheap shrimp. A six-month investigation found that suppliers to four of the world's largest global retailers (Walmart, Costco, Carrefour, and Tesco) were selling shrimp caught on "slave boats." These boats scoop up huge catches of small and infant fish and inedible species to grind into meal and feed to farmed shrimp. Since the small fish are normally eaten by larger fish, the larger fish starve; and eventually, the industry creates a dead sea.

Between 2000 and 2006, fishing was considered one of the most dangerous occupations in the United States. The average fatality rate was

115 deaths per 100,000. My father's family were commercial fishermen. I know much can go wrong on a fishing boat. Small injuries are common due to the speed of work and the sharp equipment, let alone the dangers of a rough sea. Vessel instability, large waves, and severe weather conditions cause the majority of fatal vessel disasters. Falls overboard in high seas are often not witnessed, and fishermen rarely wear flotation devices since they slow down the work. As competition becomes more intense and local fish stocks are depleted, big corporate operations take over. Boats move into deeper waters with less governmental control. Wages plunge, and the take-it-or-leave-it attitude that rules agricultural employment comes into play.

Slaughterhouses

The high speed killing of land animals is even more dangerous. No wonder we hire others to do it for us. An animal entering the front door of a slaughterhouse will exit in pieces within nineteen minutes. Pelts, organs, bones, and meat are all separated. The animal becomes a series of products. The killing and butchering that takes place on the killing floor is a dangerous world filled with sharp tools, flailing legs, and bodies of terrified animals. In 1999, more than a quarter of the 500,000 workers in the meatpacking industry suffered a job-related injury or illness. The serious injury count is five times higher than the national average, even though the industry discourages injury reports and falsifies injury data.

As in the agriculture business, it is people of color and those living on the edge of poverty who do this dangerous and psychologically deadening work. In the USA, about 38 percent of slaughterhouse and meatpacking workers were born outside US borders.

Killing for a living has other unspoken but logical consequences. Amy Fitzgerald, a criminology professor at the University of Windsor in Canada, has found a strong correlation between the presence of a large slaughterhouse and high crime rates in US communities. One might imagine that a slaughterhouse town's disproportionate population of poor working-class males might be the real cause, but Fitzgerald took that into account by comparing her data to counties with comparable populations employed in factory-like operations. In her study (released in 2007), the abattoir stood out as the factor most likely to spike crime statistics. Slaughterhouse workers, in essence, are "desensitized," and it shows in their behavior outside of work. All that killing creates a damage to the psyche of both the individual and the community.

ENVIRONMENTAL AND CULTURAL SUSTAINABILITY

We need to have a diet that is nourishing and fulfills our biological needs—one that is sustainable. As stated at the International Scientific Symposium on Biodiversity and Sustainable Diets United Against Hunger:

> Sustainable diets are those diets with low environmental impact that contribute to food and nutrition security and to healthy life for present and future generations.
>
> Sustainable diets are protective and respectful of biodiversity and ecosystems, culturally acceptable, accessible, economically fair and affordable; nutritionally adequate, safe and healthy; while optimizing natural and human resources.

"Healthy life for present and future generations" must include the health and welfare of the people who produce the food, and "optimizing human resources" does not mean exploitation. Food production reflects social and personal ethics. It demonstrates the values that we honor and our personal and social vision of a wholesome society. Slavery has far-reaching implications for our human values. How do we relate to our fellow humans? To our planet, the source of our being? What is the true cost of what we eat?

The dollars we pay for our food is not its true cost. Aside from tax money used to subsidize meat and dairy production, many of the foods that are commonly used are produced on the back of human misery. In a practical example of the rules of ecology, the foods that cause the greatest environmental and social damage most often contribute to disease.

LET THEM EAT CAKE

The impact of the modern diet on the health of the poor is another example of collateral damage. Financial inequity leads to inequalities in people's diets, which in turn leads to poor health. Lower-income families must naturally buy cheaper foods, and so they have a diet generally high in fat and sugar and very low in fruits and vegetables. Of course, the outcome is higher rates of obesity, dental caries, and all the major killer diseases.

False Ads

The "modern malnutrition" pattern that dominates in America and the United Kingdom is undoubtedly exacerbated by celebrities advertising soft drinks and sports organizations creating a false link between fast foods, athletics, and cultural prestige. The McDonald's and Coca-Cola organizations are long-time sponsors of the Olympics.

It began in 1968 when the American athletes were so stressed by the lack of junk food that McDonald's airlifted burgers to them in France. McDonald's became official sponsors in 1976. Coca-Cola claims the following: "We help people lead active healthy lifestyles through the beverage options we produce, the nutritional information we provide, and our support of programs that encourage active healthy living." The athletes in the ads bear little resemblance to the average customer. This deceit, and the ever-present branding, helps convince us that the products are healthy.

Adhering to the Social Norm

Habits that reflect the social norm become part of our behavior unconsciously, and we tend to assume that they are benign. Challenging these habits can be seen as an attack on the society that created them. If I suggest that soft drinks are a poor food choice and your father used to take you out for a soda as a treat, is that an attack on your father? These issues are particularly resonant with dietary change since diet is so closely linked to family and culture.

When I began to change my diet, I noticed that, for some people, my food choices became an irritant. I think something about my eating was placing me "outside" the party; I was being a killjoy. It reminded me of when my father tried to stop drinking and his drinking buddies would say, "Oh, come on. We'll just have a beer." They missed their friend sharing the ritual of group drunkenness. They resented his sobriety. Food and drink are social bonding agents and a reflection of shared beliefs. Unraveling these social bonds is possible, but it is not easy.

If eating an unhealthy diet is celebrated, trendy, "normal," or even associated with patriotism, people will continue their unhealthy eating without pause. The food industry relies on the appeal of junk food, with its addictive flavoring agents, to replace regional and traditional foods. The goal is to sell us identical burgers or chicken bits, whether in New Delhi or New York. In 1977, Ray Kroc, the McDonald's marketing wizard, said, "We cannot trust some people who are nonconformists . . . we will make conformists of them in a hurry." His dream has come true. The McDonald's income from its franchises is bigger than the economy of Ecuador. It is the largest distributor of children's toys in the world and operates over thirty-three thousand stores worldwide.

Fast Food Chains

Fast-food chains target the poor. The poor want inexpensive, filling meals, so they are often the most vulnerable to the fast-food diet and to the diseases that go with it. We can say that poverty is no excuse for bad diet, but the price of junk food and some important physical realities cannot be ignored. Wholesome food can be made available, but it takes education and the availability of good food to make it a reality. Andrea Freeman gives an outline example of the trap that exists in many cities:

West Oakland, California, a neighborhood of 30,000 people populated primarily by African Americans and Latinos, has one supermarket and thirty-six liquor and convenience stores. The supermarket is not accessible on foot to most of the area's residents.

The convenience stores charge twice as much as grocery stores for identical items. Fast-food restaurants selling cheap and hot food appear on almost every corner. West Oakland is not unique.

The prevalence of fast food in low-income urban neighborhoods across the United States, combined with the lack of access to fresh, healthy food, contributes to an overwhelmingly disproportionate incidence of food-related death and disease among African Americans and Latinos as compared to whites. Fast food has also spread across the globe.

Is Exercise the Solution?

We regularly hear that exercise is the solution to childhood obesity. Yes, exercise is essential, but it only works in combination with a healthy diet. A 2011 meta-analysis on the relationship between diet and exercise in obese children showed that exercise was not the primary factor in weight reduction. Objectively measured, physical activity is not the key determinant of unhealthy weight gain in children; it is diet.

The food industry loves our continuing narrative about inactive children and teens. Coca-Cola is the driving force behind Global Energy Balance Network, a new campaign to shift attention from diet/sugar to exercise. Talk of "sugar taxes" have sent the soft drink industry to the gym. This ploy can always count on celebrity assistants—such as Michelle Obama or Arnold Schwarzenegger—to get the message out. Global Energy Balance Network are using the clout of their huge PR machine and spending millions of dollars funding studies to convince us that exercise, not diet, is the key to change. The mythology that Big Food is getting behind public health is always appealing to politicians.

Is Heredity or the Environment the Culprit?

According to Professor Marion Nestle of New York University, an expert on the politics of food, "The Global Energy Balance Network is nothing but a front group for Coca-Cola. Coca-Cola's agenda here is very clear: Get these researchers to confuse the science and deflect attention from dietary intake." It works. Politicians can stay away from meaningful food regulations since it appears that industry is "volunteering" to improve health.

We prefer to ignore the Standard American Diet as a cause for obesity and illness. A report by the Academy of Child and Adolescent Psychiatry says that heredity and environment play the key roles in determining a child's risk of becoming overweight or obese. A careful reading of the report shows that if one of a child's parents is obese, then there is a 50 percent chance that the child will be obese; when both parents are obese, the child has an 80 percent chance of being obese. But they go on to say that there is no proven genetic link discovered as yet, and that *environment* really means the food they eat. So we have to assume that children learn bad eating habits from their parents and are not biologically programmed. What an insight!

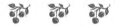

All food must be grown, raised, harvested, or processed and sent to market. At every stage of the food chain, there are opportunities for abuse and exploitation of the workers who produce the food and the consumers who purchase it. Only a dramatic change in personal food consumption will bring the radical change the world needs.

There is a willful ignorance about the way our food is produced and the harm it causes to society at large. It is essential that the study of nutrition includes the actual cost in terms of environmental and cultural sacrifice to bring down the price at the cash register. This awareness calls out to be addressed urgently given the pervasively ill effects that our food choices create. It requires that we create an ethical standard for nutrition.

An important aspect of this emerging ethic is the issue of our cultural obsession with using animals as an essential source of food. The science is certainly clear. The environmental impact of the habit is undeniable and yet we stubbornly hold on to this barbaric custom.

11

$\mathscr{R}$eaping What You Sow

I t is now a recognized fact that human activity has changed the environment dramatically since before recorded history. Those changes have never been of benefit to the web of life commonly referred to as the biosphere. It would be easy to say that we were formerly unaware of the damage we have done. The past damage was done over long periods of time, and it escaped our attention; it may be comforting for us to think that. It is certainly not the case now.

Over the past sixty years, the chorus of voices raising the warnings about our destructive habits have grown from a murmur to a roar. We have reached the point where our combined actions can be calculated on a global scale with a high degree of accuracy. The evidence is not good.

Whether we measure the effect of human actions on changing the climate, turning the seas to acid, contaminating the air we breathe, or causing the extinction of other forms of life, we are being faced with our capacity for devastation. Our actions form a pattern that is dangerous to ignore. To use a storybook comparison, we are killing the goose that lays the golden eggs.

We pretend that the problems are too complex to be addressed by individuals. Our faith lies in the hope that the solution is in a new technology or a fabulist political agreement. This is exactly what those who profit from the carnage want us to do. We once again see the strategy of confusion to delay constructive action.

In the first sentence of this book, I mentioned the estimated 8.7 million species of animal life that we share this planet with. They all have a place in the great puzzle of natural process on Earth. We should take note that every year, we are losing more species. In fact, the rate of disappearance of animal and plant life has accelerated to the point where many scientists are calling our present era the "Sixth Extinction."

The significance of this event is that previous extinctions have been driven by natural disasters, such as extreme climate activity or meteor impact. This dramatic disappearance of both plant and animal life is a direct result of human activity. Over the last 11,000 years we have over hunted animals, over fished the seas and rivers, and polluted and destroyed almost every aspect of the natural world. It is this "Anthropocene Extinction" that most represents our attitude regarding nature— our only home. Our willful ignorance of the facts does not make them go away, even in a post-truth culture driven by "alternative facts."

Food is our direct biological link to the environment, but that bond goes beyond the physical relationship. What we choose to eat reflects the ways that we perceive that connection. Our cultural and emotional attitudes are reflected by what's on our plate when we sit down to eat. There is no better example of our muddled thinking about nature than our attitudes about animals.

In previous chapters, I have tried to illustrate some of the ways that our modern diets produce disease and environmental and social damage. But what of the harm to the psyche? The choices we make in life either move us toward a deeper understanding of ourselves and the world we live in or they don't. If we desire an improved world and our choices are aligned with making that world a reality, we can make change.

Great forward-thinking people in both the modern and ancient world—such as Coretta Scott King, Albert Einstein, George Bernard Shaw, Louisa May Alcott, Leonardo da Vinci, Plato, and Ralph Waldo Emerson—have seen the moral disconnect involved in eating animals. As Albert Schweitzer said, "Until he extends the circle of his compassion to all living things, man will not himself find peace." Creating a commensal relationship with nature demands that we develop a complete regard for all life. What was once seen as the product of an excessively tender sensibility has now emerged as a critical issue.

ANIMALS AS THINGS

Many American and British people are repulsed by the idea that people in China, Korea, or other parts of the world eat dogs. The practice is called a barbaric habit and uncivilized. Horsemeat is consumed in France, Belgium, and Hungary, as well as in Mongolia and Japan. The English-speaking world is horrified—these are our pets!

In 2013, when horsemeat was found in supermarket beef patties, there was outrage. In some cases, the meat patties were 100 percent horsemeat. The legal issue was that it illustrated the difficulty involved in tracing the origin of any meat product. There was no health concern; the horsemeat would have actually been healthier than beef from a standard nutritional point of view. The public concern was that they were *horses!*

We domesticate cats and dogs to provide amusement and companionship. Foxes, minks, rabbits, and chinchilla are raised so that we can remove their skin and use their fur. We would not eat a fox; we would only wear it. We pull the feathers out of geese because they can keep us warm in a jacket with a collar made of coyote fur. We have decided that some animals are off-limits for eating, and others are OK.

Most people would agree that the killing of wild, rare, and endangered animals is wrong. It is not wrong to put them in cages with concrete floors, behind bars, or in confined spaces. Putting them in a zoo is OK; it's educational. African elephants in the wild may require up to 24 square miles as a "home range." This is considered a healthy habitat. A captive elephant in a zoo may be given two or three acres if lucky. A trained bear kept in a cage to dress up and ride a bike would have ten to twenty square miles to roam in a healthy environment. She would also hibernate through the winter. This would be like letting you live in your bedroom closet for the rest of your life. So much for entertainment, but what about the animals we raise in order to eat?

EATING ANIMALS

Science has acknowledged that all animal products are unnecessary and indeed damaging to good health, as well as bringing about the suffering of animals and environmental destruction. Our only rationale for eating these foods is pleasure. Our taste for fat and blood drives our desire. We are killing 60 to 70 billion land animals each year (estimated to double by 2050) to feed this craving.

The number of aquatic creatures killed defies counting and can only be measured by tonnage, but a conservative estimate is well over one trillion sea creatures every year. In 2016, one New England boat owner was indicted of twenty-seven counts of fraud for cheating on the allowable catch to the tune of 800,000 lb. of excess fish above the limit. That's simply one case; it is easy to imagine what that total becomes where there is little or no supervision, or the authorities simply turn a blind eye.

We might imagine that, with increased awareness about both the health and environmental consequences of this slaughter, we would stop. But we don't. We might imagine that we would never kill without a valid reason, and yet we do. What stops us?

I have taught and offered health counseling in over twenty "developed" countries. When I ask people to describe their diets, they commonly respond, "I eat a traditional diet." All their imagined "traditional" diets include meat and/or dairy foods. They are seen to be an important part of the social fabric. Celebrations and holidays are routinely associated with eating animals.

Americans fire up the grill on the Fourth of July and eat hamburgers, a food that would be very alien to the Founding Fathers. In Ireland, Easter somehow requires a baked ham or lamb. Every year, the president of the United States "pardons" an individual turkey brought to the White House by the National Turkey Foundation. (No one has yet identified the specific crime the turkey is being pardoned for.) The turkey is saved to live another day while its brothers and sisters are in the oven. Forty-six million turkeys are eaten every Thanksgiving in America. Tradition?

As with any habit, tradition should be assessed as either improving or diminishing the quality of individual and social life. Some traditions fill an important need and are worth retaining; others certainly outlive their use or may simply be based on ignorance. It doesn't make sense to retain a tradition through misplaced nostalgia. We can love our grandparents and still leave many of their prejudices and beliefs in the past.

Karma is subtle. There is perhaps no single act that more clearly illustrates our distance from nature than killing in order to enjoy specific foods. When we do that, we put ourselves outside the vibrant community of life that surrounds us. We cannot pretend that our food choices are simply a personal matter anymore than it is a personal issue if we dump garbage in the local well.

Each meal has very real effects on the lives of people around the world, on the environment, biodiversity, and the climate that are not taken into account when biting into a piece of meat.

WHEN KARMA COMES CALLING

When we ignore the laws of nature and moral considerations, the results are disastrous. Some of the results are very direct and concrete. I am not talking about punishment from angry spirits here—only karma.

When we force chickens, cattle, and pigs into cramped and crowded quarters, they breed new strains of viruses that jump species. Viruses do not simply drop from the sky; they require an environment that suits their needs. Bird flu (avian flu) breeds in the unhealthy, overpopulated environment of factory farms. Bird flu is lethal and easily jumps species. Two of every three people it infects die. These diseases are a direct result of our abuse of animals. There is no free lunch in nature.

Infectious diseases that start in animals and can be naturally transmitted to humans are called zoonosis. It is estimated that 61 percent of all known pathogens that infect humans are zoonosis, including many serious diseases, such as the Ebola virus disease, salmonellosis, and influenza. We know factory farming presents both direct and indirect health challenges to us all. Even if we were only focused on the direct effect on human health, we should be worried. These diseases are a direct result of the sicknesses we impose on the animals that live in captivity. Millions of pigs, chickens, cows, and, increasingly, farmed fish not only suffer but live in an environment that makes them ill and diseased. Even those who do not care about the welfare of animals are not excited about eating diseased animals.

THE MILK STORY

Some imagine dairy cows contently grazing in green fields. It is an image that often features in television advertisements. These ads are designed to make us feel that the cows are happy to share their milk with us. The cheese, milk, and ice cream are a cheerful gift willingly given. I remember a company that advertised their milk as coming from "contented cows." Nothing could be further from the truth.

Dairy cows are artificially inseminated and made pregnant. They give birth and are milked for up to ten months, including during their next enforced pregnancy. After being raped and confined, their children are then taken away so that their milk is not wasted on the animal it is intended for.

Anyone who has lived near a dairy farm knows the sound of a mother cow howling in anguish when her calf is taken away so that we can use her milk as a product rather than let it serve its natural purpose. It comes as a big shock to many people that cows have feelings and that they express them so clearly. Female calves are kept for future use, and males are most likely sent away for veal processing or killed.

One outcome of this unnatural condition of constant milking is mastitis, which is responsible for one in six cow deaths on American dairy farms. The disease is reflected in the quality of the milk through an increase in somatic cells. Somatic cell counts in milk are referred to as abnormal. When a cow has mastitis, up to 90 percent of the somatic cells in the milk may be neutrophils, the inflammatory cells that form pus. We don't want to consider this when we order our cappuccino or spread butter on our toast. And whether the cow was pasture-grazed, lived in a private shed with a heater and listened to classical music, or was the product of a cattle factory—she is still abused, and she is still slaughtered when her usefulness is done.

Since the animals are kept in confined and cramped conditions, viral infection is constant. In the USA, roughly 29 million pounds of antibiotics—about 80 percent of the country's total antibiotics used—are added to animal feed yearly. This contributes to the rise of resistant bacteria, making it harder to treat both animal and human illnesses. Karma!

The conditions in factory farms and feedlots around the world are horror shows of inhumanity. There is no question that the animals are tortured. They feel the fear, and they feel the pain. We want to persuade ourselves that they are unfeeling, but we know that isn't true. Our "man the hunter" mythology, speciesism, and desire for a tasty treat distorts our finer human qualities.

Previous chapters apply an ecological and social ethic to nutrition that includes, but expands beyond, physical health. But the issues around meat-eating not only span the health and environmental impacts of the food we eat but permeate our collective psyche. The ethics of eating animals were historically addressed as part of a philosophical or spiritual inquiry. The quest to live in balance with the laws of nature is important in human social development.

THE MORALITY OF ANIMALS FOR FOOD

Pythagoras (580–495 BC), the Greek philosopher and mathematician, is often referred to as the earliest vegetarian voice in the West; but vegetarian traditions, for economic as well as religious reasons, certainly predate him. There is evidence that meat-eating was debated in ancient Egyptian, Jewish, and Greek traditions. The Essenes, a Jewish ascetic sect in Palestine (200 BC to 200 AD), avoided all animal food as part of their desire to respect the laws of God. They are widely believed to be the authors of the Dead Sea Scrolls and are an important influence on early Christianity.

There were formal regulations on eating meat in the Hindu, Buddhist, and Shinto religions of the Far East. In Japan, there were several instances where meat eating of any kind was made illegal. The Buddhist empress Koken decreed that no animal was to be killed throughout the year of 752. Rice supplies were made available for the fishermen who would lose their livelihood. Religious strictures, however well-intentioned, have never passed the test of time. There has always been theological wiggle room and special dispensations. Except for extreme ascetic sects, avoiding meat has not caught on for any significant time. Colin Spencer, in the *Heretic's Feast*, suggests that this may be due to religion wanting to remain within the social norm. Belief in the invisible virtues of faith seem to trump the everyday proof of these virtues.

DOES LIFE REALLY MATTER?

Life is mysterious and undefinable. It distinguishes animals and plants from inorganic matter. It transcends the chemical reactions that form its physical foundation. Life can change and adapt to its environments in ways that serve its growth and development. Living things are complex and highly organized in structure.

Life evolves through the process of adaptation and reproduction. Human life is still evolving. We *Homo sapiens* have only been around for about two hundred thousand years. What we will become in the future depends on how we learn to relate to each other, and the diversity of life around and within us.

The two kinds of "life as we know it" are plants and animals. Plants make their own food from basic elements found in the soil, air, and sunlight. They are autotrophic; they produce organic compounds such as fats, carbohydrates, and proteins from simple inorganic substances. They are usually rooted to one place.

Animals depend on plants for food, either directly or indirectly through the plant's position at the base of the food chain. Plants can respond to environmental change and even communicate with each other, but they do not have the developed nervous systems of animals. They are reactive, not responsive.

Sentience

One of the qualities that develops with a nervous system is "sentience." Eighteenth century philosophers used the concept to distinguish between the capacity to think and to feel. We see it as the ability to experience sensations. We sentient creatures have an emotional life. We can feel fear and pain. We can suffer. We can play and feel affection. Anyone who has spent even a short time around animals knows that they share these experiences with us. Even if you have only viewed animals on-screen, you will have seen them display concern and compassion for each other. They share these traits with us and do not simply live to please us or for our amusement and use.

Even those of us who live in a world with little animal contact have seen animals exhibit altruistic qualities on the internet. A video of the "hero dog" who saves an injured dog on the highway had over 1.5 million views; over 8 million have watched a group of adult elephants helping an elephant calf recover after it collapses; 300,000 viewed a monkey working for twenty minutes to revive another who was injured by touching an electric rail at a train station in India. This monkey shakes the injured companion, submerges it in water, and slaps it till it regains consciousness and can walk away. Perhaps we know of friends or neighbors who have witnessed dogs grieving for a lost "owner."

Anthropocentrism

The concept of anthropocentrism—which suggests that human beings are the most important life-form on the planet—is as outdated as the idea that the sun revolves around the Earth. To justify our abuse of animals, we put humankind at the pinnacle of life on Earth and make mere objects of other life-forms. This attitude lies at the root of many human problems. Killing other sentient creatures diminishes us. It is a childish attempt to place ourselves outside and above the web of life.

In 2012, a prominent international group of cognitive neuroscientists, neuropharmacologists, neurophysiologists, neuroanatomists, and computational neuroscientists gathered at the University of Cambridge and produced the defining document on nonhuman sentience.

The absence of a neocortex does not appear to preclude an organism from experiencing affective states. Convergent evidence indicates that nonhuman animals have the neuroanatomical, neurochemical, and neurophysiological substrates of conscious states, along with the capacity to exhibit intentional behaviors. Consequently, the weight of evidence indicates that humans are not unique in possessing the neurological substrates that generate consciousness. Nonhuman animals, including all mammals and birds and many other creatures, including octopuses, also possess these neurological substrates.

Simply because the nervous system is organized differently does not mean that there is no consciousness.

We struggle in vain to construct a rationale for our actions. We cite science, culture, and even God as dictating our use and abuse of our fellow beings. These attempts all fall short of convincing because of one central issue—animals are sentient, and our treatment of them is unjust. Our actions are simply based on sensory and emotional drives, they are not informed by logic, science, or compassion. These beliefs stay with us because they are supported by the vast animal slaughter industries, outdated science, and our own stubborn refusal to change.

We have a tendency to separate from other forms of life and even from humans who bear different traits than ourselves. This creation of "the other" is an issue that poisons the bone and marrow of humanity. It is a trait that is foundational to all forms of discrimination—be it sexual, racial, religious, or any move to diminish the value of another because of their perceived difference. Our attitudes toward animals are not dissimilar.

Animal slavery and abuse is implemented on a colossal scale so that this massive execution can be economical. When animals are "things," they can be owned and used as the owner sees fit. Endless campaigning to "improve" the abuse and refine the killing do not change the basic facts. Many animal welfare organizations are inspired by supposed "improvements" in animal comfort within the meat, dairy, and poultry industries. These "smoke and mirror" changes are the exact strategies used by the processed-food business when replacing one fat with another or one sugar with a chemical or replacement. It sounds more natural but is fundamentally the same or even worse. Take the case of chickens and their cages.

CAGE-FREE AND HAPPY COWS

The term "cage-free" may conjure up visions of chickens roaming in open space, but there is no open space when up to a hundred thousand chickens are kept in a large warehouse. True, there are no small cages— only one giant one. "Free range" calls up grassy fields, but if it simply means there are a few doors to the outside; it makes no difference. Some occupants will work their way outside but most will never visit the barren ground surrounding their confinement. These are marketing ploys to simply make consumers feel more comfortable with the exploitation and pain imposed upon a living sentient creature.

Do concepts such as "happy cows," "grass-fed beef," or "wild-caught fish" make sense? The animal industry is actually willing to make small improvements to buffer the larger issue of consumption. Remember the power of confusion to buffer reform. The improved and "superior quality products" can be sold at a premium and help cushion the bottom line. Smart business executives have even discovered that many of the so-called animal welfare moves are good from an economic point of view.

Animal Welfare

I am aware that many feel that anything we can do to relieve the pain, enclosure, or abuse of the animals we use for food is a good thing. It is an empty argument. Either we accept that animals are sentient or we don't. This industry is not driven by a need, it is important that we remember that. The science is clear. The sacrifice of life is merely a desire. The principles of honoring life do not inhabit many gray zones. The only way to stop the killing machine is to stop consuming the products. Without consumers the killing stops.

The idea of pampering animals before slaughtering them only helps the humans involved feel more virtuous. A former killing-floor manager gave the following account: "The worst thing, worse than the physical danger, is the emotional toll. . . . Pigs down on the kill floor have come up and nuzzled me like a puppy. Two minutes later, I had to kill them—beat them to death with a pipe. I can't care." By viewing the animal as a product, or as the "other," we lose our ability to care. That our dinner could be friendly and "nuzzle us" makes us uneasy. Every "baby step" improvement means that the marketing of an animal life as a product becomes more accepted, not less.

Several modern authors have broached the issue of veganism. Perhaps Jonathan Safran Foer's book, *Eating Animals*, raised the most comment. He acknowledges that when we eat animals, we reject our own animal existence. He also addresses the secrecy that protects the public sensibility from the slaughter. But he believes that the real issue is animal welfare: we should be concerned with their "rights" before we kill them. How strange that we agree that animals are sentient, so they deserve the rights, *before we kill them*. The single and most basic right is the right to life.

Foodie Culture

Since Mr. Foer is a well-regarded modern novelist, his book was enthusiastically embraced, disregarding his muddled thinking. He has said that he has been "uncertain about how I felt [about eating meat]" for a long time. With the birth of his first child, he was inspired with "an urgency because I would have to make decisions on his behalf." It seems that he is still unable to make a decision, or rather that he has made a moral compromise that makes him comfortable.

These sentiments have washed over to the new universe of the "foodie" culture, who claim that radical change is too difficult or even antisocial. They want a trendy dietary adaptation that takes into account the "real world." They only want to be outsiders if it is fashionable. They ignore the simple fact that if you are to be healthy in a sick society, your behavior will always be outside the norm. Personal ethics are not serious if they are moderated to gain social approval. These attitudes undermine the serious issues involving nutrition and make dietary reform an elitist project.

Cognitive Dissonance

Other authors, too, such as Michael Pollan, author of the *Omnivore's Dilemma*, claim intellectual understanding and connection with a deeper instinct drives human hunger for flesh. He promotes the idea that we are programmed to eat flesh; we can't help ourselves. Pollan describes killing a pig as thrilling but admits that "part of me pities him too."

How sad that humans have no power over the urge to kill. This smug attitude tries to claim the modern fusion of intellectual insight and street smarts. In reality, it is simply the voice of cognitive dissonance. We want to be seen to love our animal friends but eat them too.

The "pity" says it all. The death of the animal is a regrettable situation, but that is simply because they had the bad fortune to not be born human. It speaks to a mythology that we are driven by passions that we can identify but are powerless to change. We don't like it, but we must kill. Man stands alone, exalted as the king of beasts, and he must exhibit power and control over lesser species. This is the same attitude that allows us to destroy the environment and be the melancholy assassins of life on planet Earth.

I love animals. But I'm not willing to sacrifice my happiness for theirs. I understand the meat industry notoriously mistreats their livestock, but as a consumer, I make conscious choices to lessen my negative effect on the animal community.

I would say that a conscious choice would be the morally consistent one: stop the killing. These are the same sentiments as those that feel global warming will be solved if we all install energy efficient light-bulbs. We could substitute the name of any racial group into that sentence in place of animals and hear the language of colonial masters and slaveholders.

Peter Singer, the author of *Animal Liberation,* has inspired many to investigate the plight of factory-farmed animals. He is a hero to many vegans and animal welfare promoters. Yet his is also a mixed message. He advocates keeping animals comfortable before killing them.

> The vegan diet, especially buying organically produced plant foods, does solve more of the ethical problems about eating than any other. But I admit that it is not for everyone, and it will take a long time before it becomes widespread. So I don't want to give the impression that it is the only thing one can do to eat ethically. Just avoiding factory-farmed products is a big step in the right direction, even if you continue to eat a moderate quantity of organically produced, pasture-raised animal products.

His position is one that is pleasing to many in the food industry. All that is needed is to change the feed, provide a little more space, and pass any increased cost to the consumer. Relativism is the best way to win friends and influence people. This attitude is growing rapidly and means that only the wealthy can eat good food.

True belief that something is an important moral stance is never concerned with how long it will take to become mainstream. This is the same attitude that slows progress in many areas of social change, from reducing the amount of sugar in soft drinks to putting modest targets for greenhouse gases. If something is dangerous to the health of all or ethically disreputable, we must not try to hedge our bets. We cannot effect significant social change unless we are personally willing to be that change. Our vaunted ability to solve problems should be more than up to the task.

This is not difficult. We can be healthy, we can be active, we can cook enjoyable food, and we can live a full life and still live by our principles. This should also apply to any abuse of animals, including the use of animals for laboratory experiments or testing cosmetics.

VALUE AND UTILITY

In 1970, I met a young doctor and his wife in Istanbul, and they invited me to join them in the long drive to Ankara. The doctor was visiting a well-known surgeon at a university hospital in Ankara, and I joined them in a visit to the university laboratory. It was the weekend, and the research unit was almost empty.

It was suggested that I wander around for twenty minutes while they took care of some business. Instead of going down to the lobby I decided to take my own tour. As I walked down the long hallways, I began to feel uneasy. The sound of high-pitched screaming was coming from somewhere in the distance. It sounded like a child in extreme pain. I made a turn and was faced with lines of cages stacked several feet high containing live rabbits.

The rabbits were all shaking, their eyes were enlarged, and some were making the screams and squealing I had heard. The rabbits had no room to move and were in a state of panic. I could not walk the full length of the hall. I retreated back to the hotel. That evening, it was explained to me that surgery students would open the rabbits up and sever and splice an artery, racing against the clock, to master a particular heart operation. The rabbits were then discarded. The fact that this torture was being done to treat a disease that could be prevented was not interesting to my travel companions; in fact, they were more than a little insulted that I would question the procedure. But using animals for experimentation is monstrous, no matter how they are used. In 1981 Dr. Irwin Bross, a former director of the Sloan-Kettering Cancer Research Institute stated:

> The uselessness of most of the animal model studies is less well known. For example, the discovery of chemotherapeutic agents for the treatment of human cancer is widely heralded as a triumph due to use of animal model systems. However, here again, these exaggerated claims are coming from or are endorsed by the same people who get the federal dollars for animal research. There is little, if any, factual evidence that would support these claims. Practically all of the chemotherapeutic agents which are of value in the treatment of human cancer were found in a clinical context rather than in animal studies.

Karma is not punishment. If we jump off a cliff, expecting to fly, our death is the penalty for ignorance, not the intervention of an angry god. Nature is self-correcting. James Lovelock demonstrated some of the wonderful adaptive aspects that the planet has. He also warned that human action could overwhelm those very mechanisms. His predictions of climate change were ignored, and now we see the results. Eating animals is a dominant part of climate change. It is universally agreed that the most serious deforestation takes place in service of feeding animals for slaughter and that animal waste is a major contributor to water pollution. Serious questions arise for me when any environmentalist insists on eating animal products.

Some say that meat-eating stimulated the growth of our large brain, and some say cooking did. Either way, we have to ask if a big brain is an advantage if you don't use it. Our biological evolution happened as a result of cooperation and adaptability, not brute strength. If weakness because of a meat deficiency is troubling, the list of elite vegan athletes should provide comfort.

EATING ANIMALS AND MAGICAL THINKING

Magical thinking has found a new home in the resistance to veganism. When cognitive dissonance raises its uncomfortable head, many proceed directly to the land of make-believe for relief. One escape hatch I have been aware of over the years has recently come to the surface again. I call it "romancing the kill."

A recent example of this is from Jason Mark, the editor of *Sierra*, the journal of the respected environmental organization the Sierra Club. Mark has written an editorial called "Toward a Moral Case for Meat Eating." I am sure many of their members celebrated this reprieve with a sigh of relief. No more worries about killing animals; it's all part of a mindful return to a long-forgotten past when humans and animals shared the planet in harmony.

In Mark's fantasy land, "the conscientious carnivore can re-establish our moral obligations to the other species with whom we share this planet." This obligation is fulfilled by using appreciation and respecting the animals that we kill for their sacrifice. It is the "thoughts and prayers" approach. This view, however strange you may think it, is not unique; it may even have a specific origin in modern American poetry.

One of the most respected poets of the American West is Gary Snyder. Snyder is an excellent and unique poet. His work is grounded in his Buddhism and environmentalism and study of Native American tradition. He is a folk hero for many. For decades, he has rebelled against what he considers the puritan aspects of vegetarianism and veganism. This is a sample of his ideas about eating animals: "If we do eat meat, it is the life, the bounce, the swish, of a great alert being with keen ears and lovely eyes, with four square feet and a huge beating heart that we eat, let us not deceive ourselves. We too will be offerings—we are all edible." In other words, it is poetic killing. This is the magic of taking on the spirit of what we eat. If we don't eat animals, we lose our animal spirit, our vitality. I wonder if gorillas or elephants miss that "bounce and swish," being herbaceous.

The environmental movement, on a whole, is caught between wanting to clean up the environment and putting a halt to polluting technologies and a desire to not give much up. It is often the work of entitled and affluent men and women with great ideas and emotional turmoil but who are still figuring out how to rationalize the SUV in the driveway or give up the artisanal cheese. The attitudes of many environmentalists is a thinly disguised speciesism. A desire to honor the mindless beasts and to treat them "humanely"—but not to stop using them for decoration, food, or entertainment. Often it is a romantic urge to be a hunter-gatherer or, as a Native American called them, "weekend Indians."

The simple fact—that the most effective action that an individual can make in daily life to halt climate change is to stop using animal products—is irritating to many. This is particularly true when the imagery of hunter-gatherer people strongly influences the "eco-minded." Tribal people have an iconic value to environmentalists for good reason.

Hunter-gatherers had a unique and powerful relationship with the environment. Their lives depended on understanding the habits and migration patterns of animals, the signs of seasonal change, and the burden of material goods. They lived lightly on the earth and represent a simpler way of living for many. Having respect for those indigenous cultures is one thing; romanticizing them and using them as a model for modern living is absurd. There are two types of evolution: biological and cultural.

I doubt that anyone would argue that there is further biological change on the horizon. In fact, there is a good case to be made for the observation that we may be devolving as a species. Cultural evolution is the only path to improvement and even survival. This process is only possible through the creation of a revolutionary secular morality. Veganism is a key part of that evolution.

Mark says, "By eating animals, we can remind ourselves of our animal natures. That recognition of our corporeal reality—the fact that we are flesh and blood and bones and skin, each of us ever on the way to very likely an unpleasant end—can, like few other things, keep us connected to the living earth." Quite frankly, this is sentimental nonsense. If he wants to recognize the reality that he is flesh and blood, all he needs to do is slam his finger in the car door.

He goes on to say that the connection between the shepherd and the sheep is based on reciprocal debts. "It is an exchange in which the sheep receives security (and the possibility of a longer life, though one capped by slaughter) and the shepherd receives sustenance. This might be confirmation bias talking, but I think such a relationship goes deeper than the eating of a broccoli spear." I would say that this appreciation of "reciprocal debts" does not show a deeper relationship with food but exactly how shallow this ecology really is. Animals who are raised on farms have a much shorter life span that they would in the wild.

It is not common knowledge the way we cut the life short of all the animals we raise for our pleasure. I have never seen anyone who doesn't laugh when watching lambs play in the field. They would have a natural life of 12 to 14 years, but they are killed when 6 to 8 months old. Dairy cows are expected to live 15 to 20 years but will only survive 4 years when expected to produce consistently till they are of no use and killed. Chickens raised for meat will only last 5 to 7 weeks. They could live up to 8 years. Male chicks produced by the egg industry are "destroyed" within the day of their hatching, they are not economically viable. Our lust for meat is satisfied by eating the babies of other species.

THE MODERN VEGAN REVOLUTION

Modern veganism is a secular phenomenon. Most vegans see the ethical issues as a simple respect of life. Since the publication in 1906 of the

Jungle by Upton Sinclair, the American public has had a queasy relationship with the meat industry. Periodic television exposés and documentary movies that show the inhumane treatment of animals have moved many to consider a new nutritional ethic. But a total cessation of eating animal-sourced foods must be adopted for effective results. This is clearly stated by Professor Gary Francione:

> If you are a feminist and are not a vegan, you are ignoring the exploitation of female nonhumans and the commodification of their reproductive processes, as well as the destruction of their relationship with their babies;
>
> If you are an environmentalist and not a vegan, you are ignoring the undeniable fact that animal agriculture is an ecological disaster;
>
> If you embrace nonviolence but are not a vegan, then words of nonviolence come out of your mouth as the products of torture and death go into it;
>
> If you claim to love animals but you are eating them or products made from them, or otherwise consuming them, you see loving as consistent with harming that which you claim to love.

Professor Gary Francione and Anna Charlton created the Rutgers Animal Rights Law Clinic to research and develop a legal framework for the rights of animals. Francione is the Board of Governors Distinguished Professor of Law and the Nicholas B. Katzenbach Scholar of Law and Philosophy at Rutgers University School of Law. His partner, Charlton, is an attorney and adjunct professor at Rutgers. The pair are somewhat controversial in the animal rights debate, firmly adopting a vegan approach consistent with the ethic that animals deserve every respect as living, sentient creatures. They have compiled six principles that define the "abolitionist" approach to animal rights. This list defines a clear vision of a commensal relationship with the animal kingdom.

- Abolitionists maintain that all sentient beings, human or nonhuman, have one right—the basic right not to be treated as the property of others.

- Abolitionists maintain that our recognition of this one basic right means that we must abolish, and not merely regulate, institutionalized animal exploitation, and that abolitionists should not support welfare reform campaigns or single-issue campaigns.

- Abolitionists maintain that veganism is a moral baseline and that creative, nonviolent vegan education must be the cornerstone of rational animal rights advocacy.

- The Abolitionist Approach links the moral status of nonhumans with sentience alone and not with any other cognitive characteristic; all sentient beings are equal for the purpose of not being used exclusively as a resource.

- Abolitionists reject all forms of human discrimination, including racism, sexism, heterosexism, ageism, ableism, and classism—just as they reject speciesism.

- Abolitionists recognize the principle of nonviolence as a core principle of the animal rights movement.

In recent decades, radical diversions from the norm drove the biggest social revolutions, as well as revolutions in nutrition and health care. Those revolutions successfully broke through the barriers of imagined tradition, nutritional mythology, and corporate food abuses to open up a healthier, more sustainable approach to food. When we align our personal habits to the greater good, and to our love for the environment, we can create a healthy world.

A MACROBIOTIC VIEW OF VEGANISM

In Chapter Seven, I outlined some of the unique aspects of macrobiotic philosophy as applied to nutrition. The practical application of these principles changed over the centuries and continues to do so. Some of the adaptations have reflected practical changes due to experience, some as a response to new discoveries in nutritional science or inclusion of Western dietary traditions, and some merely as personal preferences.

Macrobiotics is a grassroots phenomenon, and there is only a loose affiliation between teaching centers; there is no "governing body." The only attempts at defining the macrobiotic diet as a template were the

Macrobiotic Standard Diet (referred to in Chapter Seven) and later adjustments by Michio Kushi in the form of a food pyramid.

These templates were useful as a guide for many people starting the diet but often became overly limiting or influenced by the desire to gain popular acceptance. An example of the latter was the addition of white-meat fish "once or twice a week" as an option. My observation is that this was simply added to make the program seem less extreme at the time and certainly not due to any nutritional requirement. The macrobiotic diet used in the 1960s featured a broad range of vegetable-quality foods and no meat, dairy, eggs, or sugar. There were no nutritional problems, and fish was seen as a "binge" (not essential and used for pleasure).

The fact is that both Oshawa and Kushi referred to the consumption of any animal foods as inferior. Oshawa stated, "Depending upon adequate sources of food, the vegetable is normal, logical, and sure. The opposite, or carnivore way, is speculative." Basically, this is advice that eating animals is allowed only when there is nothing else available. Other examples are mentioned in Sylvia Ruth Gray's essay "Eating Animals."

It is ironic that when nutritional science now acknowledges the value of plant-based diets, some macrobiotic teachers are saying that meat should be added to the diet. The answer to this contradiction lies in understanding the underlying aim of macrobiotic practice, which is balance with the world we live in. That balance is a macro effect, it includes both the internal and external factors that are expressed as health.

Macrobiotics is animated by the desire to create a healthy human ecology. This means that our thoughts and actions contribute to personal, social, and environmental health. The use of animals as a food source is clearly not an option for these goals. Macrobiotic principles mirror the leading edge of nutritional science, the wisdom of traditional approaches to diet, and the realities of modern social and environmental concerns.

A senior devil gives a junior devil the following advice in the *Screwtape Letters* by C. S. Lewis: "The safest road to hell is the gradual one—the gentle slope, soft underfoot, without sudden turnings, without milestones, without signposts." In other words, the road to hell is not only paved with what appear to be good intentions, it is also devoid of making really difficult decisions.

In our quest to reimagine nutrition and our move away from the disaster or the modern diet, the default setting is to look for someone or something to blame. There are plenty of villains out there, both real and imagined. Greedy business bosses, crooked politicians, industrial polluters, god's will, the astrological forecast, or our position on the Aztec calendar. But what about us? Are we victims of a cruel world? The answer is no. We are the perpetrators.

It is nature and most specifically the animal kingdom that has suffered by our mistaken ideas. We are the ones that choose what we eat. The good news is that we can change all the damage done to all of nature very simply. Yes, there are other causes of environmental and social health issues but animal agriculture, the production of animals for meat, dairy, eggs and even fish farms are foundational.

What is known is—if we stopped eating animals and using animal products, the world would be a better and healthier place for us and future generations. The question is why don't we just do that?

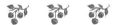

There is a great little saying that I understand comes to us from the wonderful world of investment finance. Having "skin in the game" means that you actually put in some of your own money before advising others to invest. It means that you share personal risk in a project. You are not on the side-lines cheering, you are not an observer, you are a participant. Being a vegan means you have "skin in the game" of ecological renewal; you are serious.

To create a diet based on ecological and ethical principles is not very difficult. It is a non-violent way of eating, it is inexpensive, and productive of good health. There are a few simple principles that are helpful in guiding us toward that goal. These principles will be found in the next chapter.

PART FOUR

The Road Ahead

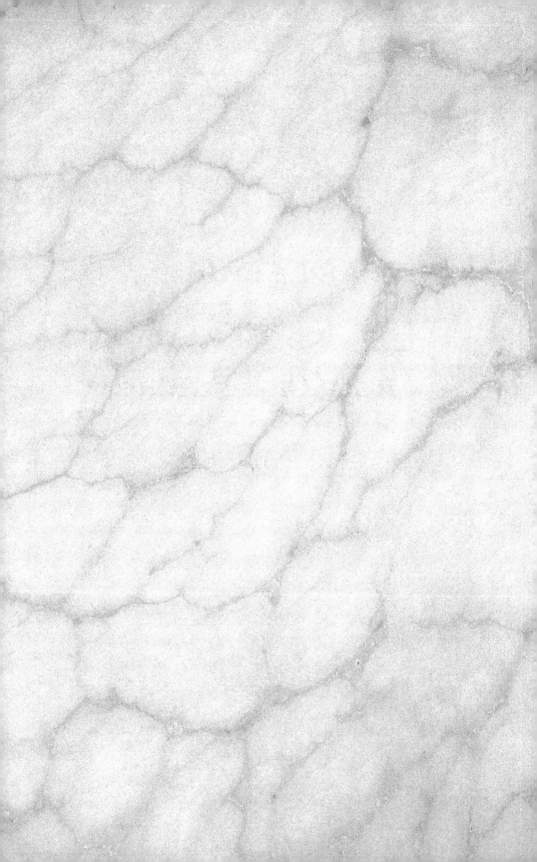

12

$\mathcal{T}$he Human Ecology Diet—What We Need

N ew superfoods or diet programs or studies often show that eating a particular food will change your life. And of course, the "new thing" is not always the best thing.

Creating a healthy way of eating is not a science project. It is seldom the lack of a single nutrient that creates health issues. Poverty is the chief cause of malnutrition. In the West, excessive consumption of fat, animal protein, and simple sugars are the major causes of dietary-related disease. The focus on single nutrients (such as, vitamin C, iron, and roughage) generally causes unfounded fears and anxiety. Our focus should be on the whole profile of a healthy diet. This approach does not mean we neglect nutritional science; it simply means that science provides us with a useful checklist to assess our overall food choices.

Even when studies indicate a benefit from consuming a particular food or a specific nutrient, those nutrients must always be considered as only a small part of the whole health profile. One isolated feature of a lifestyle usually implies other factors that may not be studied. If we were studying the health benefits of a vegan diet compared to fast-food consumption, should we take into consideration the fact that vegans don't usually smoke? If we study a population that is overweight, we are sure to find that those people don't exercise very much. Is the lack of exercise a cause of the weight, or is the weight the cause of the lack of exercise?

Macrobiotic dietary principles have been constantly developing over the past six decades through the experience of practitioners and the thousands of individuals and families who apply this way of eating in their daily life.

PRINCIPLES OF A MACROBIOTIC DIET

The philosophy of Asian medicine and folk medicine as practiced in China and Japan form the inspiration for macrobiotic practice. These concepts reflect physical, environmental, and social observations for a period of over 5,000 years. On the surface the philosophy bears little relationship to Western nutritional science, yet the conclusions are remarkably similar.

Macrobiotics is a way of understanding the effects of different foods and making choices according to individual and social needs. Michio Kushi developed the *Macrobiotic Standard Diet* in the early 1980's with assistance from myself, Edward Esko, William Spear, and Murray Snyder.

The standard diet was presented to offer a general model of macrobiotic eating. The model was helpful to the growing number of people seeking help with their health who were dealing with cancer, heart disease, and a variety of serious illnesses.

Since macrobiotics is not a set diet but a "philosophy of eating" it has fostered a variety of interpretations over the past decades. Teachers and health counselors now recommend an assortment of dietary practices. In some cases, it has become difficult to identify specifically what the term "macrobiotic" really means. This is especially true from country to country. I have labeled the diet described in this book as "The Human Ecology Diet" so that there is complete clarity.

My approach is firmly based on macrobiotic principles but also reflects personal experience in my work, the newest discoveries in nutritional science, ecological concerns, and vegan ethics. I want to be clear with my intentions. I believe that the diet as described here is an accurate application of the guiding philosophy as applied to present environmental and social conditions.

The foods listed below are the "all-time greats"—the "golden oldies" of nutrition. They are the nutrients that provide the building blocks for human nutrition. They contribute most to energy, strength, and longer life.

As you might expect, the food list includes the foods that reduce digestive stress, do not provoke inflammation, provide the best range of both macro- and micronutrients, and are most effective in disease prevention. There are five essential nutrients that form the foundation of good nutrition: carbohydrates, proteins, fats, vitamins, minerals, and water.

CARBOHYDRATES

The body runs on carbohydrates; they are our main source of energy and are especially important for brain function. Glucose is the primary fuel for all the cellular functions of the body, and brain activities use about 20 percent of the glucose we consume.

Carbohydrates can be referred to as starches or sugars. When people hear the words *starch* or *sugar,* many run for cover. But the main problem is the way we process and refine our carbohydrates.

Refined vs Unrefined

What we mostly define as sugar is the most refined product. It enters the system quickly since it does not need to be broken down. The refinement process strips away essential nutrients from the whole food, leaving only the sweet center. These sugars are the type we find in candy, soft drinks, and many common snack and food items.

Commercial flour products are also a refined form of starches. These are longer molecular chains of sugars that require more digestion. The most refined, the white flours, are also stripped of essential nutrients. These refined carbohydrates are found in noodles, breakfast cereals, cakes, muffins, and even diet puddings and desserts. These fragmented foods have a propensity to make people put on weight and can cause trouble by spiking blood sugar or by causing intestinal disorders.

Unrefined carbohydrates are whole cereal grains, wholemeal breads and pastas, potatoes, sweet potatoes, beans, most root vegetables, winter squashes, and fruits. These are all sources of healthy sugars or starches. These sugars are healthy because they digest slowly and are not stripped of the fiber, minerals, or vitamins that slow down the absorption of the sugars and complement their metabolism (the chemical process by which energy is released for use). In their whole form, they provide a healthy medium for the gut biome.

Dietary charlatans often promote confusion about carbohydrates by misidentifying the idea that "carbs" are a poor choice in a healthy diet with little or no distinction regarding processing. The best sources for sugars are in the form of the complex carbohydrates found in natural whole foods. The more refined the sugar, the more damaging it is to health. Common refined sugars are listed on food labels. Sucrose, glucose, dextrose, fructose, maltose, and lactose are fundamentally all the same and should be avoided. Products such as agave, honey, and coconut sugar are often touted as superior forms of sweetener but in my opinion are very similar to those listed above.

I prefer rice or barley malt as the best choices for sweeteners because their taste is more complimentary to plant based foods and they do have a small amount of buffering agents as well increased mineral and vitamin content. Maple syrup can sometimes be used for special occasions. The bottom line is that all refined sugars should be used seldom and sparingly. It is best to focus on the unrefined whole foods.

Our Main Fuel Source

Carbohydrates are your body's main fuel source. During digestion, sugars and starches are broken down into simple sugars. They're then absorbed into your bloodstream, where they're known as blood sugar (blood glucose). From there, glucose enters your body's cells with the help of insulin. Extra glucose is stored in your liver, muscles, and other cells in the form of glycogen, or it is converted to fat.

The mythologies regarding weight gain and carbohydrate consumption are related to the overconsumption of refined products. One needs to look no further than the cultures that rely on cereal grains as their main food to see the absurdity of the weight gain claim. It is highly refined sugars that flood the bloodstream, creating an excess of glucose that is then converted to fat for storage.

The carbohydrate debate is almost entirely driven by the issue of weight loss. Certainly, severe weight loss can be achieved by avoiding all carbohydrates. But low- or no-carb diets count on the body burning stored fats to produce energy, which will create a condition called ketosis. This is where the body starts using its protein as an energy source. Ketosis will produce weight loss, but it will also damage the kidneys and the liver.

Dietary Fiber

Significantly, eating grains, beans, and vegetables provides us with fiber. Dietary fiber is a carbohydrate that humans (and some animals) do not absorb completely. The two subcategories of fiber are insoluble and soluble. Insoluble dietary fiber consists mainly of cellulose that is indigestible by humans, because humans do not have the required enzymes to break it down. Soluble dietary fiber comprises a variety of oligosaccharides, resistant starches, and other carbohydrates that dissolve or gelatinize in water. Many of these soluble fibers can be fermented or partially fermented by microbes in the human digestive system to produce short-chain fatty acids that are absorbed, therefore providing us with some calories.

Fiber provides bulk in the intestines, and insoluble fiber especially stimulates peristalsis—the rhythmic muscular contractions of the intestines that move food along the digestive tract. Some soluble fibers produce a highly viscous solution gel, which slows the movement of food through the intestines. This is important for getting complete digestion.

PROTEIN

If carbohydrates are the fuel for the body, protein is the form. Protein is responsible for creating the foundation for cells and tissues, as well as controlling biochemical reactions and aiding the immune system. Proteins regulate metabolism and hormones, repair damaged cells, and create new ones. Protein is found in all vegetable foods to varying degrees.

The human body is about 60 percent water, 16 percent protein, 16 percent fat, and 6 percent minerals. Carbohydrate is only about 1 percent at any given moment, and vitamins, minerals, and the like exist in only minute amounts. These ratios can change quite a bit from person to person and are influenced by environmental as well as some genetic factors. Some body cells are slow to renew, and others are replaced very quickly.

Red blood cells can live for 120 days, and connective tissue can live for years, while the epithelial cells that line the digestive system and blood vessels are replaced every three or four days. The body is in a constant process of breaking down and building up.

Process of Breaking Down and Building Up Protein

A common image is that by eating muscle, we gain muscle, because muscle is constituted from protein. This assumption would be similar to saying that if I read great novels, I am sure to produce a best seller. The concept of "complete protein" only means that an animal has composed the components of the protein already. Where do cows or sheep get their complete protein? They make it of course. All the foods we eat are broken into their primary elements and then reconstructed according to the specific needs of our body.

When we take in the protein of a cow, a chicken, or a pig, it has already been made into the cow, chicken, or pig. We will have to break it down in order to create a human out of it. Imagine choosing between a huge mansion that we can break apart to build a home of our own or simply given all the supplies we need to build to our own specifications. Some will accuse me of cheating with this example since both animal and vegetable proteins need to be broken down. But vegetable protein is easier to disassemble, digest, and more bioavailable.

Amino Acids

The basic elements of protein are the amino acids; they are the building blocks we need to create human protein. We can make some of these, and we acquire some through our food. Those we cannot make are called the "essential amino acids." Out of the twenty amino acids required for good health, eight are considered essential. They must be present in our diet, although they don't need to be in a single food.

As an example, beans are high in the amino acid lysine and low in methionine, while grains have complementary strengths and weaknesses. This means if beans and rice are eaten over the course of a day (or even several days), their amino acids will supplement each other and provide a higher quality protein than either would alone. All vegetables contain protein as well as nuts, fruits, grains, and beans. Traditional cultures have recognized these complementary relationships for thousands of years. The grain-and-bean combination is near universal in agrarian societies around the world.

FATS

Fats are organic compounds that are only soluble in alcohol (not water). They are also called lipids. They are stored in the body as energy reserves and are important components of cell membranes. In a healthy person, they have a protective function in cell structure. This is especially true in terms of epithelial cells. As with carbohydrates and proteins, there is massive confusion about the use of fats in a healthy diet.

Fats are needed to help you absorb vitamins A, D, E, and K—the "fat-soluble vitamins." Fat also fills your fat cells and insulates your body to help keep you warm. Fats are made of a variety of fatty acids. The need for fatty acids is very small. According to the National Academy of Sciences, our daily requirement could be achieved by one-fourth teaspoon of fatty acids a day. Using seeds, nuts, grains, and beans easily exceed the minimum requirement.

In the past, the focus on "good" and "bad" fats and cholesterol pushed perceptions to a "micro" approach to the issue. The main use of fats has traditionally been its thermogenic functions in cold climates—to produce warmth and insulation or to make food tastier (fats trigger a dopamine response and provide "mouth-feel"). The high-fat diet is tasty.

The old good/bad scale had to do with saturated and unsaturated fats. The "good" fats were generally identified as those unsaturated fats generally found in plant foods. These fats are found in olives, soy, corn, nuts, seeds, and (in lesser amounts) in grains and some vegetables. When extracted from their source, they remain liquid at room temperature. The general use for these fats is in the form of vegetable oils. These oils are either chemically processed from the plant or, more rarely, pressed. They are a highly processed product.

For many years, the focus was on reducing animal fats, such as butter, cheese, milk, and fatty cuts of meat. So the food industry began to produce "low-fat" products and to promote the use of vegetable oils. The trick was to use the "healthy" vegetable oils and still retain the taste, or "mouth feel," of animal fats. The end result was the same.

Common sense tells us that sticky, fatty foods are difficult to digest and make sticky, fatty blood. It makes no difference if the excess fat is from a vegetable oil or an animal. Remember, these are highly processed and wasteful foods. It can take between three and twelve kilograms of olives to produce one litre of oil, depending on the quality of the oil. A tablespoon of oil would be the oil of 40 olives. What a treat.

Essential Fatty Acids

Our bodies easily use unsaturated fats when taken in the form of plant foods. The digestive process extracts the fats to be used according to our body's needs. The body creates all the fatty acids required for good health—with two exceptions. These two are called the essential fatty acids. They are linoleic acid (an unsaturated omega-6 fatty acid) and alpha-linolenic acid (a polyunsaturated omega-3 fatty acid), and both are sourced from plants. It appears that it is an imbalance between these two fatty acids that causes the most health challenges from fat.

The Western diet may have a ratio of anywhere from sixteen to fifty times the omega-6 fatty acid to one part omega-3. This is one of the primary features of the modern fast-food diet. A healthy plant-based diet is estimated to be around 1:1. Diets high in omega-6 are associated with inflammation and a variety of serious health issues, such as heart disease, stroke, diabetes, and Crohn's disease. Fried foods, baked goods, fast foods, and processed foods are sources of high levels of omega-6.

Saturated Fats vs Unsaturated Fats

The other concern with fats is the level of "saturation." Saturation describes the physical composition of the fats, which are usually divided into saturated or unsaturated. The highest concentration of saturated fats is in red meat, butter, cheese, and all milk products. Some vegetable oils, such as coconut oil and palm oil, also have high concentrations of saturated fats. These two vegetable oils—common in so-called "healthy" products—mimic the texture of butter or other animal fats. Yes, they are vegan, and palatable—but present the same problems as any saturated fat.

The connection between saturated fats and blood cholesterol is well known. Cholesterol is manufactured in the body, and it can also be consumed directly in animal-derived foods. It is used in the structure of cell walls and in making up digestive bile acids in the intestine, the constructing of hormones, and allowing the body to produce vitamin D. But if the body's needs are exceeded, the waxy cholesterol can build up and create deposits in the arteries, causing blockages.

Saturated fats contribute to LDL, or "bad" cholesterol, as opposed to unsaturated fats (found in good-quality vegetable foods), which contribute to HDL, or "good" cholesterol. The distinction between the good and bad cholesterol has to do with whether it can be returned to the liver and excreted easily or is more apt to be stored.

Trans Fats

If saturated fats are "bad," then trans fats are "very bad." Trans fats are the manufactured fats used primarily in food processing. They are basically vegetable-sourced fats that have been saturated to mimic the mouth feel and processing qualities of animal fats. These fats increase inflammation and all disease risks. The manufacture of these foods is achieved by taking unsaturated vegetable fats and then saturating them (making them solid). Their invention was largely a result of attempting to create a market replacement for animal fats. The plan to increase vegetable oil consumption worked. Americans in 2000 consumed, on average, 3.6 times more salad and cooking oil than they did in the 1950s.

Even the use of better-quality vegetable oil in a healthy diet is questionable. Oil causes our red blood cells to clump together, limiting their ability to absorb and deliver oxygen to our cells. This clumping, sometimes referred to as sludging, then leads to a slowing down of our blood flow. Studies have shown that our blood flow decreases by over 30 percent for the four hours following a fatty meal.

The real issue here is not how much animal-sourced fat we need but if we need it at all. The arguments about primitives who ate (or indigenous people who still eat) significant amounts of fat in their diet are disingenuous. They most often disregard the ecological habitat, the unavailability of sufficient nutritious vegetable food, and the short life span of these people. Mythologies abound regarding the lack of heart disease among the Inuit or the Maasai people of Africa. All the original observations on the Maasai were done without adequate information on their diet. One fact was undoubted though. The Maasai walk about twelve miles a day, certainly a massive energy output compared to a modern person's. Regarding the Inuit, who live above the Arctic Circle, the prevailing mythology has been that they were free of heart disease and yet ate a diet very high in animal protein and fat. This turns out to be false. Based on actual autopsies, they show the opposite. It turns out that they have a very high rate of heart disease, as well as very poor bone health.

VITAMINS

Vitamins are essential nutrients that we need in small amounts on a regular basis. They are organic chemical compounds that are understood to be either ineffectively produced by the body or that cannot be synthesized. They must be obtained through the diet. There are thirteen vitamins needed for good health. There are two primary categories of vitamins: fat-soluble and water-soluble.

Fat-soluble vitamins are stored in fatty tissues of the body and the liver. They are easier to store than water-soluble ones and can stay in the body as reserves for days, some of them for months. They are absorbed through the intestinal lining with the help of fats. Vitamins A, D, E, and K are fat-soluble. Vitamins D and K can be made by the body.

Water-soluble vitamins are quickly excreted in the urine. Because of this, they do not stay in the body, and they need to be replaced more often than fat-soluble vitamins. Vitamins C and all the B vitamins are water-soluble.

- **Vitamin A is a fat-soluble vitamin.** It is associated with good vision and support for a healthy immune system. It is found in carrots, broccoli, sweet potato, kale, collard greens, apricot, cantaloupe, and melon.

- **Vitamin B is a water-soluble vitamin.** Deficiencies can cause beriberi. It is found in sunflower seeds, brown rice, whole-grain rye, asparagus, kale, cauliflower, potatoes, and oranges.

- **Vitamin B2 is water-soluble.** Deficiency may cause ariboflavinosis, a protein deficiency disease that can cause dysfunction of the liver. It is usually found in poorer populations. The vitamin is found in asparagus, bananas, persimmons, okra, chard, and green beans.

- **Vitamin B3 is water-soluble.** Deficiency may cause pellagra, an illness that causes diarrhea, mental disturbance, and dermatitis. Good sources include avocados, dates, tomatoes, leafy vegetables, broccoli, carrots, sweet potatoes, asparagus, nuts, whole grains, legumes, mushrooms, and brewer's yeast.

- **Vitamin B5 is water-soluble.** Deficiency may cause "pins and needles." Good sources include whole grains (unhulled only), broccoli, and avocados.

- **Vitamin B6 is water-soluble.** Deficiencies may cause anemia and peripheral neuropathy (damage to parts of the nervous system other than the brain and spinal cord). Good sources include whole grains, banana, vegetables, and nuts.

- **Vitamin B7 is water-soluble.** Deficiency may cause dermatitis or enteritis (inflammation of the intestine). It is found in some vegetables.

- **Vitamin B9 is water-soluble.** Deficiency during pregnancy is linked to birth defects. Good sources include leafy vegetables, legumes, and sunflower seeds. Several fruits and beer contain moderate amounts.

- **Vitamin B12 is water-soluble.** It is the only real concern among essential nutrients for vegans. Deficiency may cause megaloblastic anemia (a condition where bone marrow produces abnormal and immature red blood cells). B12 is made by bacteria found in the soil and in the intestines of animals. Although humans produce B12 in the digestive tract, it is not reabsorbed to any significant degree. The vitamin can be stored in the body for a period of up to six years in adults.

   B12 is crucial for a healthy nervous system, and a chronic lack can eventually cause neurological symptoms. It is recommended that we consume B12 in food such as fortified yeast extracts or nutritional yeast. Vegans are advised to take supplements.

   In some early macrobiotic teachings, there are claims that some fermented foods (such as miso and tempeh) contain significant amounts of B12; however, this would only be true if the products were made in an environment where there was a high rate of bacterial "contamination" not found in modern production. Our obsession with protecting ourselves from harmful bacteria means that we do not profit from the direct or indirect benefits of the helpful ones.

It's easy to see why we might imagine B12 to be in foods that do not, in fact, contain it. There can be B12 analogues that do not function as B12 but resemble it in analysis. Some of them are harmless, but some attach to receptor sites and block them. Homemade tempeh, for example, would quite probably have B12, and so might home-fermented vegetables such as sauerkraut. Unique among vegetable-sourced foods, nori seaweed has been shown to have significant amounts of active B12.

Many vegans rely on fortified breakfast cereals, fortified soy milk, and fortified meat analogues to provide themselves with adequate B12. This can certainly solve the nutrition issue; however, I prefer to take a simple supplement and avoid "fortified" foods. Specific brands of nutritional yeast are a reliable source. Be sure to check the nutrition facts label or the ingredient list to ensure you are receiving the active form of vitamin B12 (called cobalamin or cyanocobalamin). It is easy to find vegan B12 supplements on the internet or in grocery stores in developed countries.

A small number of people with no obvious reliable source of B12 appear to avoid clinical deficiency for twenty years or more. The issue needs more study, but supplementing is the best clear route. B12 is the only vitamin that is not recognized as being reliably supplied from a varied whole-food, plant-based diet with plenty of fruits and vegetables, together with exposure to the sun. Vegans using supplements are less likely to suffer from B12 deficiency than those eating a meat-centered American diet, with up to 6 percent of that population suffering from a deficiency.

- **Vitamin C is water-soluble.** Vitamin C is a powerful antioxidant that can help prevent cell damage. Deficiency may cause megaloblastic anemia, which is related to DNA damage in the creation of red blood cells. Good sources include fruits and vegetables. Cooking destroys vitamin C, so a small amount of raw vegetables or fruits daily is a good idea.

- **Vitamin D is fat-soluble.** It aids in the absorption of calcium for strong bones. Deficiency may cause rickets and osteomalacia (softening of the bones). It is produced in the skin after exposure to UV (ultraviolet) light from the sun or artificial sources. Also found in mushrooms. This is particularly true if the mushrooms are placed in a sunny location with the "gills" exposed.

- **Vitamin E is fat-soluble and is an antioxidant.** Deficiency is uncommon but may cause hemolytic anemia in newborns (a condition where blood cells are destroyed and removed from the blood too early). Good sources include almonds, avocados, nuts, leafy green vegetables, wheat germ, and whole grains.

- **Vitamin K is fat-soluble and is essential for blood clotting.** Deficiency may cause bleeding diathesis (an unusual susceptibility to bleeding). Good sources include leafy green vegetables, avocados, kiwifruits, and parsley.

MINERALS

The minerals in our diet are important for building strong bones and teeth, blood, skin, hair, and muscle, and for nerve function and metabolic processes. We need quite large quantities of calcium, chloride, magnesium, phosphorus, potassium, sodium, and sulfur. Other minerals—commonly referred to as "trace minerals"— are essential in tiny amounts. They include iron, nickel, zinc, iodine, selenium, silicon, chromium, molybdenum, vanadium, and cobalt. Eating a diverse plant-based diet (such as the Human Ecology Diet) ensures sufficient consumption of all these elements.

- **Potassium, sodium, calcium, magnesium, and chloride are electrolytes that can be found in almost all vegetables.** Electrolytes are substances that conduct electrical charges when dissolved in water. They regulate nerve and muscle functions, body pH, blood pressure, and the rebuilding of damaged tissue. An imbalance in electrolyte levels can lead to either weak muscles or muscles that contract too severely.

- **Calcium and phosphorus help support bone health.** They are abundantly available in a wide variety of plant-based foods, including kale and collard greens, sweet potatoes, broccoli, carrots, chickpeas, and almost every other kind of legume, whole grain, and fruit.

- **Iron is essential for blood production.** About 70 percent of your body's iron is found in the red blood cells (hemoglobin) of your blood and in muscle cells (called myoglobin). Hemoglobin carries oxygen from the lungs to the cells and tissues. Iron is found in green leafy vegetables, beans, and dried fruits.

- **Zinc ensures your immune system functions well.** It plays a role in cell division, cell growth, wound healing, and the breakdown of carbohydrates. Zinc is also needed for cognition and the senses of smell and taste.

- **Iodine is needed to make thyroid hormones, which control the body's metabolism and are essential for proper bone and brain development during pregnancy and infancy.** Iodine deficiency is a global public health concern, affecting nearly one-third of people worldwide. Because iodine content varies widely in soil, it's unreliable in plant foods. Sea vegetables can either have a lot of iodine or very little. Good sources are navy beans, potatoes with skin, and dried sea vegetables. Dulse and kelp are the best sources.

Minerals are found in abundance in all green vegetables—which, of course, are a part of any healthy diet. All of the fifty-six minerals essential for human health are present in sea vegetables (including calcium, magnesium potassium, iodine, iron, and zinc) along with important trace elements, such as selenium (often lacking in land vegetables due to soil demineralization). The minerals in sea vegetables exist in a chelated colloidal form that makes them easier to digest and utilize. Although usually consumed in small amounts, they can be an important part of a healthy diet.

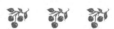

It is worth remembering that these minerals and vitamins are only needed in fairly small amounts but are essential. That is why a diverse diet is essential. Some people will experiment with vegan foods and find two or three things they enjoy and stay with those. That will undermine health in the long run. That is why we suggest that grains, beans, a variety of both green and root vegetables, nuts, seeds and fruits all be taken on a regular basis.

Do not become enchanted with the popular habit of juicing and making smoothies as a regular meal. Good health is dependent on a healthy gut biome. Plenty of fibre is known to help the biome thrive. Chewing whole foods aids digestion and creates more satisfaction in the long run. Cooking grains, beans and many vegetables is important since it softens the fibre and makes the nutrients more available as well as providing a broader range of taste. The next chapter will review the major food groups, provide a little history about them in common use, and suggest some ratios for using them.

13

*H*uman Ecology Diet— Where We Get What We Need

T he focus of nutritional studies has shifted away from food and toward the individual components of food. While that is an interesting study, it has not really informed the debate as to what a healthy diet looks like. What foods do we need in order to get the proper balance of nutrients? It turns out that the answer is not a mystery.

If we look at the leading edge of nutritional science, we see that there is little disagreement. Certainly, there are conflicts with those who stubbornly defend the past, who have a vested interest in a particular product, or who refuse to believe that the foods they love can possibly be harmful, but these arguments are superficial and unimportant. If we apply the considerations in previous chapters regarding personal health, social justice, environmental concerns, and ethical considerations, we arrive at the Human Ecology Diet. It is a simple approach and contains all the foods essential for personal, social, and environmental well-being. The ingredients are not "superfoods" packed with powerful and mysterious micronutrients. In fact, a healthy diet is more a fusion of traditional diets from around the world with the simple considerations of ecological and economic realities taken into account.

The food groups listed below are not based exclusively on botanical classifications but, rather, on the groupings that are familiar to a person shopping in a local market. For a quick overview, see the inset on the following page.

The Human Ecology Diet

Use this table as a daily guide in order to benefit from the food groups and cooking condiments that suit your personal needs. The foods and condiments listed below are the nutrients that supply you with the building blocks for human nutrition. Use organic, seasonal, and local products when possible. Choose non-gluten products if necessary.

WHOLE CEREAL GRAINS. Consume whole cereal grains at least two meals a day

BEANS or TEMPEH. Eat cooked beans or tempeh at least one meal a day

COOKED VEGETABLES. Consume a diverse range of cooked vegetables at least two meals a day

RAW VEGETABLES or SPROUTS. Eat a smaller portion of raw vegetables or sprouts depending on the climate

FERMENTED MISO or SOY SOUP STOCK. Eat fermented miso or soy soup stock at least once a day

FERMENTED BREADS or NOODLES. Eat naturally fermented bread or noodles

SEA VEGETABLES. Add sea veggies as a condiment or side dish once a day

SEEDS AND NUTS. Include roasted seeds and nuts as a garnish or snack once a day

SEASONAL FRUIT. Eat fresh seasonal fruit at least once a day

WATER. Drink 3 to 4 glasses a day and/or tea as desired

WHOLE GRAIN

The Human Ecology Diet has cereal grain as its foundation. Taken as a group, the grains can feed more people per acre with semi-perishable food than any other food. The nourishing qualities of eating grain plus the ability to store grain for long periods of time with little spoilage have made it the most important single crop in human history. It has assured societies the capacity to survive through periods of drought or the presence of harmful pests. It was insurance against the bad times.

The nutritional profile of grain is excellent. It contains protein, vitamins, minerals, carbohydrates, fats, and fiber in a form that is easy to digest and metabolize. Grain is versatile in use and can be cooked as is, or can be made into porridge, breads, or noodles.

Unrefined Grains vs Refined Grains

In the Human Ecology Diet, when I talk about whole grains, I am always referring to unrefined cereal grains. This means that only the inedible husk has been removed. The outside shell of the grain (the cellulose) has not been broken. The grain, with this outer skin intact, is capable of being sprouted and contains the germ, the carbohydrate, and the bran. The micronutrients in the grain are protected. When the outside cellulose is removed, the process of oxidation occurs, and the grains begin to lose their nutritional value. This process is what we call refining.

As I mentioned in Chapter 2, "whole grain" on the label doesn't mean whole grain in the product. The refining process always changes the nutritional value. When the outside seal of the cellulose level is removed, oxidation begins. Aside from the loss of fiber in refined products, there is a loss of protein and antioxidants. This is an important distinction to remember because the food industry will try to fool you at every bend of the road.

Government recommendations always suggest that you increase your consumption of whole grain and then proceed to have pictures of loaves of bread and pasta and breakfast cereals. This inaccurate definition of whole grain leads consumers to choose poor-quality grain products with the idea that they are eating the healthiest option. Most of the bad press for whole grains comes from a lack of clarity between these refined products and whole grains.

It is refined flour products that cause the problems. We need to question the saying, "Best thing since sliced bread." These are products that have virtually no nutritional content, and they are usually filled with sugars, fats, and chemical agents. The commercial breads (including most "whole wheat" varieties), cookies, muffins, cakes, and pizza crusts are a nutritional nightmare mix of trans fats, refined grain, and simple sugars. These foods raise blood sugar and are difficult to digest.

Much of the confusion regarding whole-grain consumption is purposely generated by those who support a high consumption of animal-sourced foods. I consider most of this propaganda to be misleading at best and completely counterintuitive. Books like *Wheat Belly* and *Grain Brain* are poorly disguised advertisements for the Atkins diet and its many more recent incarnations, such as the Paleo diet. These low-carbohydrate diets can produce short-term weight loss but are actually dangerous as a healthy way of eating.

Phytic Acid

The issue of phytic acid in grains also became a hot topic for a short time. This is a substance found in grains and nuts and has been labelled as an "anti-nutrient." The compound binds with minerals in the body and was thought by some to cause mineral loss when eaten. The truth is that this is only a problem when consumed in great quantity as part of a nutrient-poor diet.

This compound is easily deactivated by simply cooking the grain. Soaking grain overnight, sprouting the grain, boiling, fermenting, or germinating also deactivate phytic acid and free up minerals for absorption. According to Rosane Oliviera from the University of Davis, "the consumption of whole grains in recommended amounts seems to have no adverse effect on mineral status whatsoever." Since it is a powerful antioxidant, phytic acid may be instrumental in reducing the risk of heart disease, diabetes, and obesity.

Primary Grains

Among indigenous North and South Americans, the primary grain was maize (corn) or quinoa in the high Andes, oats in the British Isles, buckwheat and barley in Europe, wheat, millet, and rice in the Near and Far East, and wheat and millet in Africa. These grains became synonymous with settled culture.

Agriculture demonstrated the shift to a commensal relationship with the environment discussed earlier. This was the capacity to intelligently farm so that the same land could be used over and over again, and people could stay in one place without completely depleting their resources. The approach of modern organic agriculture is an attempt to return back to this kind of understanding of our relationship to the environment with modern insight and without the chemical maintenance of the soil.

- **Rice has been cultivated in the Far East for nine thousand or ten thousand years, and then slowly spread into the Near East and into Europe.** Mediterranean-style cooking has incorporated rice for centuries with dishes like paella, stews, and risottos.

  This is the most nourishing grain and possibly the most delicious. Its naturally sweet taste can be enjoyed on a daily basis. For a complete meal, eat rice with a bean dish, a variety of vegetables, and fermented pickles.

  Brown rice gives you lots of fiber, vitamins and minerals, and small amounts of thiamine, riboflavin, vitamin B6, folate, and niacin. These B vitamins tend to work hand-in-hand to metabolize the energy from the foods you eat, while supporting blood-cell formation. You'll also get magnesium, phosphorus and calcium, potassium, and a small amount of sodium for fluid balance and heart functions.

- **Millet has been cultivated in the Far East for at least ten thousand years and eventually spread into Africa, where it is used still to this day.** In some cultures it is the principal food crop. In Europe it was never as popular; but as people became more used to using whole grains in their diet, it has become more mainstreamed/prominent. Some may find that lightly roasting millet before using it brings out its sweetness. Oftentimes, people use gravies or sauces on top of the millet as it can have a tendency to be a little dry. It can also be used as a porridge and is also good added into soups and stews.

  Millet is alkaline and it digests easily. The serotonin in millet is calming to your moods. Millet is a super carbohydrate with lots of fiber, and it is low in simple sugars. Magnesium in millet can help reduce the effects of migraines and heart attacks. Niacin (vitamin B3) in millet can help lower cholesterol. Scientists in Seoul, South Korea, concluded that millet may be useful in preventing cardiovascular disease.

All millet varieties show high antioxidant activity. It is an effective alkalizing agent and is the only whole grain that does not produce stomach acid, so it is a great food for those who have suffered from ulcers.

Millet is gluten-free and non-allergenic. It is a great grain for sensitive individuals, and the high protein content (15 percent) makes it a substantial addition to a vegan diet. Millet and other whole grains are a rich source of magnesium, a mineral that acts as a cofactor for more than three hundred enzymes, including enzymes involved in the body's use of glucose and insulin secretion.

- **Barley is a grain that has wonderful warming qualities when eaten, but it is usually associated with brewing and making beer.** It's a wonderful food in the colder months.

One of the most popular uses for it is, of course, to use it in soups and stews as it makes these dishes creamy and hearty. There is nothing nicer on a winter day than a barley vegetable stew. Barley has an inedible portion of husk that runs down the center of the grain. Because of this, most barley is "pearled" and thus refined. By itself, barley is a great low-fat grain chock-full of nutrients, and it is reputed to aid the body in breaking down fat.

- **Oats are similar to barley in use; rolled oats and oatmeal are the common forms, but the whole grain can be used as porridge.** Similar to barley, this is an excellent winter grain, particularly in cold and wet climates. This is due to the fact that it has more fats than other grains. Steel-cut oats (US)—also called pinhead oats, coarse oatmeal (UK), or Irish oatmeal—are groats (the inner kernel with the inedible hull removed) of whole oats that have been chopped into two or three pieces. Steel-cut oats are traditionally used to make porridge as well as oatcakes and the like.

- **Quinoa is often touted as a superfood, particularly because of its high protein content, but, interestingly, oats have more protein than quinoa.** This is a grain that thrives in a dry, high environment, such as the Andes, where it originates. It is still the principal food for many of the native people that live in those high mountain areas. It has been domesticated for over seven thousand years. Quinoa should be rinsed well before cooking to remove the outer coating—the saponin can give the grain a slightly bitter taste.

It contains high levels of protein and a nearly perfect balance of essential amino acids. The small yellow seeds turn translucent when cooked. Compared to other grains, quinoa is higher in calcium, phosphorus, magnesium, potassium, iron, copper, manganese, and zinc.

- **Corn is a grain that developed in Mesoamerica in prehistoric times.** Up to the first European landings, most Native American people on the East Coast of America, the Southwest, Mexico, and South America were living on a diet that was based around the consumption of corn, or maize. Corn can either be eaten fresh as sweet corn or ground into a meal.

- **Buckwheat has a very strong taste; however, some people (myself included) love the hearty, earthy taste.** Buckwheat is the most warming of all the grains. Its use has been traced back to very cold areas, particularly in Mongolia, Tibet, Russia, and Finland. It has been documented to be in use since about 5,000 BC, and in the Balkans it was cultivated regularly from about 4,000 BC.

  Buckwheat is actually a "pseudo cereal." It is gluten-free, making it a popular substitute for other wheat-based foods. You can use this as a grain in soups, or you can use it with sauces, but most people are familiar with it as being used in noodles or as a flour product. In whole form, it is eaten primarily as "kasha," and in noodle form as soba or as a porridge.

  Buckwheat is also high in manganese, magnesium, copper, and zinc, which are great for the immune system. It contains all eight essential amino acids, including lysine, which plays a key role in collagen production and is not produced by the human body.

- **Wheat is the most widely used of all the cereal grains.** Most of it is ground and made into flour products. Hard wheat varieties have more gluten in them and are therefore used more popularly to make both noodles and flatbreads. Wheat products are popular in almost every cuisine around the world, in one form or another, but usually used in breads.

  Wheat is rich in mineral salts, calcium, magnesium, potassium, sulfur, chlorine, arsenic, silicon, manganese, zinc, iodide, copper, vitamin B, and vitamin E. This wealth of nutrients is why wheat is often used as a cultural base or foundation of nourishment. Since there is a high gluten content in wheat, some may find it an advantage to remove wheat from the diet for a test period and see if they notice a difference.

Most problems that are experienced with wheat may be down to three factors:

1. Flour products can wreak havoc if there is poor digestion; whole grain that has not been finely ground is easier to digest. Because the bread dissolves quickly in the mouth, it is seldom chewed well and mixes with the digestive enzymes in the mouth that aid digestion.

2. Breads often contain yeast, sugars, milk, or other products that inhibit digestion or create nutritional problems.

3. The presence of excessive gluten. Modern bread and baked food production has favored very high gluten varieties of wheat. Making sourdough bread, where commercial yeast is not used, is better if you have no specific problems with bread use.

The sourdough process uses a starter that contains naturally occurring lactobacilli and yeasts. The fermentation that takes place makes the bread more digestible, needs less gluten (can be made with low-gluten varieties of grain), and does not create the lift in blood glucose that yeasted bread does.

Getting the Most From Grains

Using whole grains as the foundation of your diet is not only healthy but also economical. Grains can be cooked and stored to be re-used for up to five days. They can be reused as grain "burgers" mixed with vegetables or beans, used in soups and stews or simply heated and used with a condiment or sauce. Try and have at least one or two servings of grain a day.

BEANS

Beans are usually mentioned in relation to protein for those consuming a plant-based diet. The concept of a "first-class" or "complete" protein dies hard. This focus on meat protein as being superior deflects the issue away from the simple fact that all plants contain protein. It would be more accurate to call animal protein "secondhand" protein.

Most plants and microorganisms can synthesize all twenty of the standard amino acids that are needed. Animals, including humans, are unable to synthesize all the amino acids and so must obtain some of them from their diet. Any amino acids that are needed and cannot be synthesized are referred to as "essential" amino acids. Humans need to obtain eight amino acids exclusively from the food they eat.

Some plants contain all the essentials, including quinoa, buckwheat, soybeans, chia seeds, and hemp seeds. Combining rice with beans is one of the most popular combinations and is used in one form or another in many cultures.

The key is to consume a variety of plant foods and to include both whole grains and beans on a regular basis. This is because, while all plant foods contain some of the essential amino acids, there is only a few that contain all. Dietary diversity allows the body to construct protein as it is needed. That is why the grains and beans are part of the foundation in the Human Ecology Diet.

- **Kidney beans, being a major source of protein, provide all the basic forms of amino acids.** Studies have revealed that the darker the color of the skin of the beans, the higher the antioxidant content. They are high in fiber, magnesium, iron, and copper.

- **Adzuki beans are small and compact shiny red beans that are lower in fat and oil than other beans.** Adzuki beans are easier to digest than most beans, and in Asia, they are thought to strengthen the kidneys. They're a great source of magnesium, zinc, iron, copper, potassium, fiber, manganese, and B vitamins, such as niacin, thiamine, and riboflavin.

- **Garbanzo beans (chickpeas) have a wonderful nutty taste and creamy texture when cooked.** These are wonderful to use in bean dishes combined with sweet vegetables or corn, as well as in soups and stews. The choline in chickpeas helps with sleep, muscle movement, learning, and memory. Choline also helps to maintain the structure of cellular membranes, aids in the transmission of nerve impulses, assists in the absorption of fat, and reduces chronic inflammation.

- **Pinto beans are a very good source of cholesterol-lowering fiber, as are most other beans.** In addition to lowering cholesterol, pinto beans' high-fiber content prevents blood sugar levels from rising too rapidly after a meal, making these beans an especially good choice for individuals with diabetes, insulin resistance, or hypoglycemia.

  When combined with whole grains such as brown rice, pinto beans provide virtually fat-free, high-quality protein. But this is far from all pinto beans have to offer. Pinto beans are a very good source of folate and protein, vitamin B1, and vitamin B6, as well as the minerals copper, phosphorus, iron, magnesium, manganese, and potassium.

- **Lentils are an ancient legume that comes in many varieties, from common brown-green to red to yellow to lentils Le Puy (a tiny sweet French variety, which are great in salads).** Very high in protein and minerals and with a full-bodied, peppery taste, lentils are good in everything from stews and soups to salads and side dishes. Low in calories and high in nutrition, lentils are the perfect legume to eat in summer salads and to make delicious soups and stews for the colder months of winter.

- **Soy beans are always mentioned as the most efficient way to achieve the full complement of amino acids.** In the Far East, they have proved a life-saving crop for many centuries. There is a huge difference between the ways that soy foods have been traditionally used in Asia compared to their more recent use in the West.

  Using the Western approach to nutritional science, the soybean was recognized as a valuable source of protein but not really studied in terms of its normal dietary use. This has stimulated a commercial rush to put soy into anything and call it a "health food." Soy is now found in a variety of products, such as soy milk, soy yogurt, imitation meat products, and as a filler in many standard grocery products. It is also a popular source of feed for animals.

  Vegetarian diets and other plant-based approaches to nutrition were common in Asia, and they developed simple food technologies to create healthy foods from vegetable sources. The benefits of the soybean were prized—but only when processed, mostly through fermentation. Foods like miso paste, tempeh, soy sauce, natto, and a wide variety of soy foods were developed. These foods are unique and very valuable. The process of fermentation makes the nutrients more bioavailable. It is important to note that these foods are used in relatively small amounts in the daily diet.

Without fermentation, soy is more difficult to digest. This is especially true with children, and it should not be given to infants as a formula to replace mother's milk. This is because of the concentration of protein in these formulas. Since the baby is only getting their protein in the form of this concentrated soy, the phytoestrogens present a problem. In this concentrated form, they are several times higher than for adults who are eating soy foods.

- **Miso, for example, is a nourishing, high-energy whole food that helps maintain health and vitality.** The same enzymes that help with fermentation during the making of miso can also help with digestion of a meal that includes miso, and can even destroy substances that cause food allergies. Miso also acts like a digestive tonic, and once established in the intestine, the acid-loving bacteria (found in abundance in unpasteurized miso) promote health and stamina.

The fermentation process creates the probiotic bacteria (the "good bacteria") that your gut requires—such as lactobacilli, which has been shown to increase the availability, quantity, digestibility, and absorption of nutrients in the body. Nutritional researchers agree that—rather than specific nutrient content—it is the cultured soy medium that is responsible for fermented soy's health benefits.

Miso has long been suspected to be one of the most significant influences in the high levels of health among the Japanese. Miso is a probiotic, a living ingredient. Miso's lactic-acid bacteria help to maintain a healthy digestive system. A 2003 report that followed 21,852 Japanese women for ten years showed that eating three bowls (or more) of miso soup every day reduced breast cancer risk by one-half.

Studies report that regular miso consumption may reduce the risk of liver and breast cancer by 50 percent to 54 percent. The breast-cancer protection appears especially beneficial for postmenopausal women. In an extensive review of over one hundred experimental and epidemiological studies, the *Journal of Toxicologic Pathology* identified miso as being helpful in the suppression of cancer tumors, the lowering of blood pressure, and even resistance to radiation damage.

Obtaining adequate protein in our diet is certainly not a problem. Concentrated protein-rich foods have been made for centuries in Asia. None of them require extensive processing, and none of them taste like meat. They do not fit the bill if you are trying to pretend you still eat meat but don't want to feel somehow deprived. The food industry has taken soy in many forms and manufactured it to have "meaty" or "cheesy" flavors.

About Fake Meat

The issue of meat substitutes brings up issues that go deeper than simply the providing of a tasty treat. It speaks to our attitudes about what we eat, some potent mythologies of nutritional science, and our place in nature. They are issues that I believe are important for anyone who is vegan, macrobiotic, or would label themselves an environmentalist. For decades, the whole topic of eating animal products or to avoid them has revolved around two issues: nutritional need and pleasure. When the issue of nutritional need is debunked, the default setting is, "But I love meat." It is a sensory, emotional, and often sentimental attachment.

Since increasing numbers of people have come to the conclusion that meat is not a good choice, this decision invariably affects social and personal habits. What if you like the taste of meat? What if you like the texture of meat? What if you simply like the idea of meat? Food science is on the way to your door with a wonderful resolution to your concerns: fake meat. Pretend meat, pretend milk, and pretend cheese is flooding the marketplace.

Soy protein isolate is a favorite ingredient in artificial soy meat substitutes. Soy burgers, soy sausages, and lunch meats are mostly touted as healthy replacements for meat. The problem is that the products are made from soybeans (usually GMO) that have had all the fat removed and washed in a chemical bath or water to remove the natural sugars and fiber.

A company called Beyond Meat recently caught the eye of the

multibillionaire Bill Gates. The young entrepreneur who started the company is busy cranking out all sorts of fake meat in his factory. He outlined his idea in an interview with *Business Insider* magazine.

> Meat is well understood in terms of its core parts, as well as its architecture. Meat is basically five things: amino acids, lipids, and water, plus some trace minerals and trace carbohydrates. These are all things that are abundant in non-animal sources and in plants.

Here we are again in the "food as a chemical delivery system" world. So far, they have manufactured artificial chicken (it tastes just like chicken) and beef in his new facilities in Southern California. The prevalence of these foods is a clear indication of our addiction to "junk food." If we are concerned that the junk is either environmentally damaging or unhealthy, we simply try to make what seems to be a "healthier" junk replacement. The quality differences are often marginal, and the irony escapes us.

Another option soon coming to market is SuperMeat. This is a science-fictional product that takes animal stem cells and "grows meat muscle and fat" in the lab. The cells are placed in a "meat-growing environment," and the product is said to taste just like the real thing since it is simply artificially grown meat without being attached to any particular animal.

The Swedish Institute for Food and Biotechnology did a study on the carbon footprint of various protein-source meals. What they discovered was that a meal using peas as the major protein required a fraction of the energy required to produce the same calories as pork. When they compared peas that were processed into a "pea burger," the footprint was roughly equal to a pork-chop.

These products are being marketed as a solution to the "meat problem." But we don't have a meat problem. We have a human problem. It is a problem that goes to the source of our relationship with planet Earth. Do we feel that we need meat at some level, or do we really need to alter our thinking and accept the fact that nature provides our needs without superficial improvements? We seem determined to meddle with the laws of nature to suit invented social habits. It's good to remember that nature knows best.

Claiming a new relationship with nature and all life is revolutionary and transformative; the rejection of consumerism is part of it. It is within our power to occupy the food supply and reduce our reliance on an industry that separates us from the simple pleasures of choosing real food, local food, and foods grown in living soil. So who needs fake meat? Nobody.

- **Tempeh is a good example of a natural protein-rich food.** It is made by using a controlled fermentation process that binds hulled, cooked soybeans into a cake form. Tempeh originated in Indonesia and is still a staple there. The beans are mixed with a mold spore starter and incubated for two days. The white mycelium of the *Rhizopus* vegetable mold keeps the soybean packed together to form a sliceable cake. As a result of the fermentation process, the soy protein in tempeh becomes more digestible. Tempeh is fiber-rich and a healthy source of vegetable protein, minerals, and soy isoflavones.

  Tempeh is low in saturated fat and contains a generous source of B vitamins, iron, calcium, and lecithin, plus essential polyunsaturates, such as linoleic acids. These acids are important because they help emulsify, disperse, and eliminate cholesterol deposits and other fatty acids that frequently accumulate in and around vital organs and throughout the bloodstream.

  Tempeh is always cooked before eating; you can steam, boil, bake, or sauté it. You can enjoy it with a wide variety of grains, vegetables, or noodles, or use it in soups, salads, and sandwiches. It is a very versatile addition to a healthy diet.

- **Tofu is a staple food that has been eaten throughout Asia for the past two thousand years.** Tofu is known for its good nutritional and culinary versatility. It has a cheese-like quality and is laboriously made by curdling "milk" made from boiled soybeans with a natural coagulant. It's notorious for its bland taste, but tofu blends with and absorbs flavors from other foods. Rich in B vitamins and a vegetable protein source, tofu is often portrayed as a meat substitute. Tofu is taken traditionally with miso soup as a meal, but it's perfectly fine to use in the occasional dessert or marinated patties. Always buy a brand that is made from organic whole soy beans and nigari.

  Nigari is a naturally occurring, mineral-rich coagulant produced after removing sodium chloride from salt. The base of nigari is magnesium chloride, which is an alkalizing mineral vital for the proper functioning of the cells in our body. It also has numerous other beneficial mineral salts in abundance, such as potassium chloride and calcium chloride. Tofu is an excellent protein as it has all the eight amino acids.

Soy and Estrogen

The growing popularity of soy products has led to controversy about their health and safety. These concerns have been raised by some (again, those suggesting a diet reliant on animal protein) regarding the presence of phytoestrogens. The phytoestrogen compounds can mimic the hormone estrogen because of their similar structure, and they can inhibit the function of naturally occurring estrogen in the body.

What is seldom pointed out is that plant estrogens are a thousand times weaker than the estrogen produced in our bodies. They are only significant if they are eaten in amounts that would never be part of a normal diet. What has been shown in the bulk of soy research is that it is helpful in preventing some cancers and other serious health issues.

When using these soy foods, it is always good to read the labels and use only products that are certified organic and made with non-GMO beans.

Getting the Most From Beans

As with grains, you can store beans for several days in the fridge and recycle them. Many people actually prefer beans when recooked. Soups, stews, and casseroles are common ways of using beans. They combine well with onions, and other root vegetables as well as the squashes. It is a good idea to have beans, or bean products at least once a day. I also suggest the use of miso soup regularly several times a week.

VEGETABLES

Vegetables reflect the changing of the seasons; the different colors that that they show indicate the phytonutrients that are in the foods. A good guideline is to always try and eat any perishable food from local sources and in the season of its growth. Be particular about organic quality. The challenge is to consider these things but to make sure to get variety. This is particularly true if you live in an area where local weather, poor soil, or lack of local variety is a problem. There are hundreds of varieties of vegetables. Listed below are the general characteristics of some popular vegetable varieties.

The **CRUCIFEROUS VEGETABLES** are very important for most people living in the northern hemisphere in a four season climate. They include cabbage, broccoli, cauliflower, and curly kale. Vegetables in this particular family are best when they are cooked. They can sometimes be a little bit difficult to digest if they are not cooked well. Cabbage has been a staple food in Europe for centuries, both cooked and fermented as sauerkraut.

These vegetables are very nutrient-dense, and they are often known to have particular healing qualities, including anti-inflammatory properties. A review of 206 human studies and 22 animal studies in the *Journal of the Academy of Nutrition and Dietetics* showed a pronounced protective effect of several varieties of vegetables, including cruciferous vegetables, carrots, and allium vegetables.

Cruciferous vegetables include arugula, bok choy, broccoli, broccoli rabe, Brussels sprout, cabbage, cauliflower, Chinese cabbage, collard greens, daikon, kale, kohlrabi, radish, rutabaga, and turnips.

As discussed earlier in the section on macrobiotic classification (page 216), foods that hold their energy for a long period of time and don't wilt or dissipate very quickly are foods that are very important when the weather is cooler (or in cold weather). These foods have more warming qualities.

SQUASH is a very diverse family of vegetables that originate in the northern hemisphere in the Americas; the cultivation of food crops in both North and South America rotated around maize (corn), beans, and squash. They were sometimes referred to as the three sisters. The combination of these three foods gave people an incredibly rich and nutritionally diverse diet that sustained the native peoples of North America for centuries before the arrival of the Europeans.

They are a fantastic autumn and winter food. They can be stored for months without losing their nutritional value. They are a great source of complex carbohydrates and are very sweet to the taste, so they are very useful in cooking. Their sweetness makes them popular as vegetable dishes (cooked with beans) or even used as desserts. Because of their natural sweetness and more complex sugars, they are often used by Marlene and me for people with type 2 diabetes when switching to a Human Ecology Diet.

The **Summer Squash**—which are sometimes referred to as cucumbers in shape and consistency—are foods that don't have that particular density of nutrition, but they are cooling and best used in season when they ripen with the exception of being useful to preserve as pickles. The squash family include pumpkins, acorn squash, Hokkaido pumpkins, butternut squash, cheese pumpkins, Hubbard squash, kabocha squash, and turban squash.

Roots and Tubers are vegetables that grow below the ground. Most of the roots and tubers have been used traditionally as good sources of complex carbohydrate all over the world. They have often been used as a primary food source when climate or other environmental conditions were not favorable to growing grain. Some tubers have an even broader range of nutrients than grains. This is probably why—before grain cultivation in semitropical climates—they were the principal foods. They even have vitamins A and C.

Roots are the energy storage system of the plant. Similar to some of the other foods that we have talked about, these foods are nutritionally dense and have traditionally been considered as essentials to a healthy diet. Foods like carrots and onions, potatoes, yams, and sweet potatoes will last a long time without losing their nutritional qualities.

These vegetables include (some were listed earlier as cruciferous as well) carrots, daikon, parsley root, parsnips, beets, celeriac, radish, rutabagas, turnips, burdock, salsify, and taro. (Botanically, onion, garlic, shallots, spring onions, and leeks are alliums.) The most popular tuberous roots are sweet potatoes, yams, and potatoes.

Hearty Greens are a basic requirement for healthy eating. Some cruciferous vegetables mentioned earlier will fit into this category. If you are eating a plant-based diet, I think it is very important to have green vegetables every day. The unique concentration of nutrients in dark-green vegetables lies in the rich mix of vitamins and minerals. These greens pack a more significant punch than the salad greens we will talk about next. If you have a good seasonal balance, you are going to have a good nutritional balance. The dark-green vegetables include, but are not limited to, collards, mustard greens, turnip greens, chard, spinach, and kale. Most of these vegetables are best lightly cooked (more so with kale).

Lighter Greens (Salad Vegetables) Even when the climate is cold, people (especially those who have eaten a lot of animal fats) need some raw food. Raw foods are helpful in cleaning out the gut and dissolving fatty tissue. Have small amounts of raw food daily—but remember it's easy to eat too much of it in a cooler climate.

Whether it's pressed salads or light fresh salads, consume these cooling foods in the summertime. Varieties of lettuce, "rocket," or any of the spring greens can be eaten raw and are good to have on a daily basis.

These salad vegetables are relaxing by nature. Aside from their cooling qualities, they are an excellent source of vitamins and enzymes. We manufacture enzymes in our bodies, but it's good to get some enzymes in our diet (although many are destroyed during digestion). Eating salad vegetables or raw vegetables ensures that you get the full spectrum of foods you need.

Vegetables reflect the seasons, so let the seasons be your guide. Food is often shipped long distances, so use produce that has traveled only when local or regional supplies are inadequate.

Vegetables that are seldom cooked include arugula, endive, chicory, dandelion greens, escarole, radicchio, watercress, iceberg lettuce, Bibb lettuce, and romaine lettuce.

Fermented Vegetables are important probiotics, which are good to have in small portions daily. *Sauerkraut,* one of the most common, is easy to make. Making fresh fermented foods can really promote a healthy gut biome. There are good-quality commercial sauerkrauts on the market, but making it at home is a satisfying project.

Juicing and Sprouting are quite popular now, particularly in warmer seasons and climates. Many advocates of juicing and sprouting live in Florida or Southern California, where refreshing foods make sense.

Sprouting is a good way of having salads and that light freshness in your diet all year round. Sprouting seeds or beans is simply germinating them. You rinse seeds to clean them and then soak them for up to twelve hours (depending on the type of seed). You drain the seeds and rinse at regular intervals. As the beans germinate, the nutrients are broken down and become more available. The quality of the protein is improved, and the vitamin and fiber content is increased.

Sprouts can be used year round. Mung beans, alfalfa, broccoli seeds, and lentils are all easy to sprout. Add them to just about anything from soups to salads and grain dishes. Enzymes are the catalyst for proper food absorption. Living foods are loaded with live, active enzymes. Enzyme-rich foods boost energy, feed the cells, nourish the organs, tone the blood, regulate the bowels, and support immunity. Thus, living foods can help you beat fatigue and will make your skin glow.

Juicing has become popular as chewing has become unpopular. When you juice, notice the amount of pulp that is left behind. That pulp is part of the nutrient base of the food. Removing it challenges our digestion and wastes valuable minerals, fiber, and vitamins. Ecologically, economically, and from a health point of view, it is a wasteful process.

The **Nightshades** are a family of vegetables permeated with mythology. Nightshades include some plants with highly toxic features (such as tobacco and belladonna), and they also include potatoes and tomatoes, aubergine (eggplant), and peppers. Within that family of foods, there are chemical compounds that have a tendency to exacerbate inflammatory processes in the body.

Solanine is a toxic chemical found in members of the nightshade family, which is also known as the Solanaceae family. The chemical acts as a natural pesticide. Plants produce solanine to protect themselves from insects and fungi that attack them. Solanine and related chemicals are found in potatoes, tomatoes, eggplants, red and yellow peppers, and other nightshade plants (but not in black pepper, which belongs to a different plant group). When creating a diet for someone who suffers from a major inflammatory illness, we eliminate all nightshades. On a health maintenance diet, I suggest that they be used sparingly and to make sure they are always well cooked.

GETTING THE MOST FROM VEGETABLES

The key to vegetable consumption is variety. It is the diversity of vegetables that assure the best nutrition. Think in terms of color. A healthy plate of food usually has a variety of colors. Roots, cruciferous vegetables, leafy greens, squash, and onions vary with season and local availability but make sure of variety. Have vegetables at least twice a day and make sure to have some raw vegetables daily.

SEA VEGETABLES

In some parts of the world, sea vegetables are traditionally consumed in moderate amounts regularly, to provide a balanced intake of minerals. We normally associate their use with Japan and Korea, but they were also part of the traditional Scottish and Irish diets.

Kombu is a good source of iodine, which is necessary for proper thyroid function. Researchers in the United Kingdom found that it strengthened the gut mucus and slowed down digestion. It was also very low on the glycemic index and high in fiber. High consumption of sea vegetables (kombu) helped in the predigestion of pulses, which reduced the production of gas.

Seaweeds are low in fat, very low in calories, and rich in essential minerals, vitamins, and protein. Seaweeds are very beneficial to vegetarians and those abstaining from dairy foods because of their high levels of calcium, iron, and iodine. In addition to minerals, seaweeds contain vitamins, A, B, C, and E. All sea vegetables contain significant amounts of protein, sometimes as much as 48 percent.

The **sea vegetables** include **nori** (usually used in making sushi or as a condiment), **kombu** (used in making soup stocks or cooked with beans or vegetable stews), **wakame, arame**, and **hijiki** (used as side dishes), and **dulse** (used with vegetables, in soups, or as a condiment).

It is important to check with distributors that all sea vegetables have been harvested from clean waters and have been tested for heavy metals. The same properties that sea vegetables have for attaching themselves to toxins in the body for excretion also make it easy for them to absorb toxins in the water. This is the same as demanding organic growing for vegetables. There are many good sources, so do your homework.

Nutrients in sea vegetables cleanse the colon and improve digestion and absorption. Research shows that the sticky starch in sea vegetables can strengthen gut mucus, slow down digestion, and allow food to release its energy slowly. Sea vegetables have an antibiotic effect on harmful anaerobic bacteria. Their unique range of polysaccharides removes pollutants, toxins, and heavy metals. Sea vegetables bind heavy metals and radioactive pollutants (deletion) (present in the environment from industry and transport) and remove them from the body. Sea vegetables improve the full digestion and metabolism of nutrients from other foods, and they facilitate the formation of new cells.

Harvard University has published a paper proposing that kelp (kombu and wakame) consumption may be a factor in the lower rates of breast cancer in Japan. Research is also being done on the effects of sea vegetables as an alternative to hormone replacement therapy. Sea vegetables are very high in lignins, plant substances that become phytoestrogens in the body—meaning that they help to block the chemical estrogens that can predispose people to cancers like breast cancer. Sea vegetables have traditionally been used in Asia to treat cancer, heart disease, and thyroid problems.

Getting the Most from Sea Vegetables

Sea vegetables may be a new food in your kitchen, but you will find them a valuable addition. You don't need large quantities to have benefit. Most people who are new to using them find using wakame in soups the easiest place to start. A tablespoon a day of cooked sea vegetables is about right.

FRUIT

"Eat more fruits and vegetables." This is a familiar health message that blurs good nutrition lines in several ways. Fruit is high in sugar. This sugar (fructose) is not as disruptive to the system as the refined fructose we discussed earlier, particularly when consumed in a whole fruit, but it is still a simple form that is absorbed into the system quickly. However, at least fruit contains fiber, minerals, and vitamins, which slow down the potential negatives.

Sugar comes in several different forms: glucose, fructose, and sucrose. Glucose is the healthiest source of energy. Carbohydrates, such as those in grains and vegetables, break down into glucose, your body's main source of fuel. Fructose is the only type of sugar found in fruits. When eaten in excess, it presents health challenges similar to those of the simpler refined sugars. Given the huge difference in sugar content from fruit to fruit, it's almost impossible to suggest how much to consume. We should think carefully about our five a day.

People who cut back on all simple sugars for a month or two commonly become more sensitive to more complex forms of sugar in their food. Until then, people often do not perceive the sweetness in a carrot or in brown rice, partly because you have to chew in order for the sugars to begin breaking down. Also, the more we consume simpler forms of sugar (like fructose), the less we detect the sugars in other foods. So we need to re-educate our taste buds.

Fruits in general are very perishable—so they are best eaten fresh and in season (and local, where possible). As a general rule, tropical fruits are the highest in sugars and acid and are the most perishable. Fruits grown farther from the equator have a higher ratio of fibre to sugar so the impact on blood sugar is less. Drinking the juice of fruits is probably the worst form of consumption, since the sugars are more concentrated and the buffering agents have been removed. Sugars are also concentrated in dried fruits, so a raisin has more sugar content by weight than a grape.

Eating fruit in smaller amounts is generally a good idea. Fruit can also be cooked into purees, sauces, or baked. It makes great fillings for pies or as a smooth dessert dish. Think of fruit as a pleasure food, not an essential. There is nothing you can get from fruit that you cannot get from vegetables. It is a good idea to have fruit an hour or so after a meal, or between meals, for best digestion. Here are some non-tropical fruits: apples, strawberries, cherries, blueberries, watermelons, cantaloupes, peaches, plums, raspberries, pears, and apricots.

Getting the Most from Fruits

Do your best to focus on locally grown foods in season. When this is difficult try regional fruits from similar climate. Use fruits that are seldomly shipped long distance or not at all. Remember that dried fruits have high sugar content. Most fruit is best eaten raw, but cooking fruit is a healthy option for making fruit compote.

NUTS AND SEEDS

Seeds and nuts are an excellent source of protein and fat. When unshelled, they are easy to store for a long time. Once shelled, they are susceptible to rancidity if left at room temperature, unless preserved with salt. The oils in seeds and nuts complement grains and beans to provide the full range of amino acids needed to meet protein needs, and they also contain easily assimilated and healthy oils. They may be used as condiments with grains or vegetable dishes or roasted as a snack. Roasting nuts and seeds releases their oils, making them easier to digest.

Nuts and seeds are an excellent source of fats in a healthy vegan diet. They contain healthy mono- and polyunsaturated fats—fats that manage inflammation, maintain the normal structure of our cells, and lower cholesterol. Extensive research associates nut consumption with a lower risk of coronary heart disease (CHD).

The tree nuts—such as **Macadamia, Cashew, Brazil Nuts and Pecans** all have a fairly high fat content. Most of the fat in nuts is monounsaturated fat, as well as omega-6 and omega-3 polyunsaturated fat.

The **Walnut, Almond and Hazelnut** are native to Europe and have slightly lower fat content.

Chestnuts are used in many parts of the northern hemisphere and have the least fat of any nut; they are rich in carbohydrates and the only nut that contains vitamin C.

Peanuts have among the highest amounts of fats in this group. They are from a different botanical family than true tree nuts but are commonly thought of as a nut. They are widely used as a snack item or as an ingredient in snacks, for their oil, or as animal feed. A handful of any of the tree nuts supplies more than the daily requirement of healthy fats.

Seeds are often used as a garnish on foods, particularly with whole-grain dishes. **Pumpkins seeds, sesame seeds, sunflower seeds, chia seeds, flaxseeds, and hemp seeds** are all sources of omega oils and add flavor and variety to the diet.

Allergic Reactions

Allergic reactions to nuts principally affect young children, and these may be severe or even life-threatening. They are caused by allergenic seed storage proteins. A smaller number of people have allergic responses to seeds. Possible symptoms of these allergies are hives or swelling, trouble breathing, tightness of the throat, nausea, abdominal pain, and diarrhea. The symptoms can vary between mild to severe.

Generally, those with allergies are allergic to several foods, the most common being milk, eggs, shellfish, and wheat. Between 1997 and 2008, the number of children reported with nut allergies more than tripled. According to two 2018 studies presented at the American College of Allergy, Asthma, and Immunology's annual scientific meeting, 2 percent of children have peanut allergies. These allergies and the immune dysfunctions that lay behind them arise as a wide range of common health problems, such as eczema and respiratory complaints.

Getting the Most From Seeds and Nuts

Either roasted or raw nuts and seeds are a healthy addition to the diet as a snack or as a garnish. I usually suggest seeds over nuts as a breakfast garnish for porridge and Pumpkin and Sunflower seeds as a snack item. In our house we usually only use nuts in dessert items.

SIMPLE CONDIMENTS

In the Human Ecology Diet, we use few table condiments. Our cooking condiments are generally miso and soy sauce, herbs and spices. Some of these products contain salt, so use them sparingly or not at all, to suit your own preference.

It is a good idea to use condiments and herbs and spices in moderation. The most healthy eating should have a variety of tastes. Sometimes it is also good to splash out on extreme taste for celebration, but for the best results learn to adapt to the true taste of the foods themselves on a daily basis.

WATER

Your body needs water—it is the most common element in the human body. About 60 percent of the weight of an adult body is water. This can be altered by any number of factors, including age, general health, and the amount of fat tissue. More fat cells usually mean less water. We get water in our food and by drinking.

I am not a fan of putting exact requirements on water consumption, but it is good to drink pure water on a daily basis. It is one of the greatest facilitators of toxic discharge. Some foods are diuretics, they leach water out of the system. These include coffee, tea, carbonated drinks, alcohol, citrus fruits and tomato. Let your sense of thirst be your guide. Your urine color is a good guideline, dark urine usually indicates you need more water, very pale or clear urine may mean you are taking too much.

Make sure to do your best to avoid water in plastic bottles and in most places a simple home filter is a good idea.

TEAS AND BEVERAGES

Here is a list of some of the most popular teas used on the Human Ecology Diet. Always buy "organically grown" and "fair trade" products.

Green Tea, native to China and India, has been consumed globally for centuries. After water, tea is the most consumed beverage in the world. All types of tea (I don't include varieties, which are, in fact, infusions rather than true teas) are harvested from the same bush; the only difference is in the way the leaves have been treated. Over 78 percent of the tea consumed worldwide is black, and only about 20 percent is green tea.

Green tea is picked, allowed to wither, and then steamed. This helps the tea retain many of its nutritional components and gives it a lighter taste. Black tea is crushed and then rolled, which lowers the antioxidants but brings out a stronger taste.

Kukicha is a traditional Japanese method for processing tea, which uses both twigs and leaves. It is an excellent mild daily beverage loaded with antioxidants and is wonderful for the digestive system. You can purchase the tea in twig form or in teabags. It has very little caffeine, so it is not a stimulant.

Nettle tea is made with the leaves of the stinging nettle, which has tiny hairs on its fresh leaves that can sting the skin. Despite its rough exterior, nettle is one of nature's best remedies for an assortment of ailments—including anemia, high blood pressure, rheumatism, arthritis, coughs and colds, congestion, urinary tract infections, and kidney and bladder problems.

Chamomile tea is often recommended for people who have trouble sleeping. It has very relaxing properties. Chamomile also calms the mind and helps people relax and deal better with their stresses.

Ginger tea both stimulates and soothes the digestive system. Ginger is an energizer and stimulant. Ginger can aid people who are experiencing nausea.

The peppermint in **Peppermint tea** is a fragrant herb that makes for a soothing drink. Peppermint helps you digest foods better, and it also reduces flatulence and digestive issues. A cup of peppermint tea will ease nausea and vomiting, especially if you suffer from motion sickness. If you have heartburn, don't drink peppermint tea as this might aggravate your condition. The natural mint flavor of the herb helps to freshen your breath. It also has cooling properties and can be added to green teas or *kukicha* for a cool summer drink.

There is a common mythology that simply cutting out animal fats and protein as well as sugar will provide good health, but this is not the case. Reducing those foods that are stressful to the system is a good move. Toxic food creates sickness and good food creates health. It is not simply cutting things out; it is also what you add in.

A diverse diet, such as that described above, will stimulate the body's natural capacity to create health, increase energy, and fortify the immune system. The process needs no professional supervision; (unless you suffer from a serious health issue) it is self-directed. The only thing we require is a firm resolve to create a healthy life and the ability to learn a few new life skills. That is what I will address in this next chapter.

14

Creating a Food Ethic

Given what we know about the problems with the modern diet and the mythologies that drive nutrition, we have to ask some basic questions. What do we really need, and how do we decide? A casual glance or a serious search on the internet throws up an endless list of absolutely essential foods, many given almost mystical power to heal or harm. With so much conflicting opinion, how can there be a rational resolution to all these debates?

There are two broad and mostly conflicting camps of nutritional opinion. On one hand, there are those who either directly or indirectly support the food industry. This support is often put forward with slight concern that "eating too much" of the products on sale is not sensible, but "moderate consumption" will be just fine. When you hear a food described as fine in moderation or "as part of a healthy diet" run for the hills. Most doctors, nutritionists, and dieticians fall into this camp. They are complacent supporters of a status quo that produces disease.

GOVERNMENT SOURCES

Politicians, acting as representatives of the food industry, are complicit in the shell game of nutritional standards. The endless stream of pie charts, pyramids, and nutrient-value, color-coded labels are convenient distractions from the need for change. The fear of industry backlash outweighs any amount of science or common sense. The result is that junk food continues to prevail and healthy options become a niche market for the affluent consumer.

I am not going to credit the USA Dietary Guidelines since they are so influenced by corporate lobbies that they are redundant. These statements by Dr Walter Willett, Professor of Epidemiology and Nutrition and chair of the Department of Nutrition at Harvard University, says it all.

> The 2016 Dietary Guidelines are improved in some important ways, especially the removal of the restriction on percentage of calories from total fat and the new limit for added sugar. Unfortunately, Congress censored the Scientific Advisory Committee's conclusion that red meat consumption should be reduced for reasons of planetary health; this was within the scope of the committee because it is not possible to have food security if our food supply is not sustainable. However, the USDA went further and also censored the Scientific Advisory Committee's conclusion that consumption of red and processed meat should be reduced for health reasons.
>
> Further, the clear scientific conclusion that sugar-sweetened beverages should be reduced were also censored in the final recommendations. The rationale for the USDA to produce the final Dietary Guidelines after the report of the Scientific Advisory Committee is that they would translate the science into messages that would be clear for the American public. Instead, the report of the Scientific Committee was very clear about the adverse health effects of red and processed meat and sugar-sweetened beverages, and the USDA has engaged in censorship and obfuscation.
>
> **Clearly, these guidelines bear the hoofprints of the Cattleman's Association and the sticky fingerprints of Big Soda** [emphasis is mine]. They fail to represent the best available scientific evidence and are a disservice to the American public.

We cannot ever expect to hear a clear message from government sources regarding a healthy diet, so what about the trailblazers?

VEGAN AND NATURAL FOODS ADVOCATES

Among the popular vegan and natural foods advocates, there are some minor disagreements, but those are slowly disappearing. The Physicians Committee for Responsible Medicine says the healthy diet should contain whole grains, legumes, and beans, along with plenty of vegetables and fruits. They suggest we avoid cheese and all dairy, meat, eggs, white potatoes, white bread, sugar, and added oils, and fatty foods, such as peanut butter and avocado. OK, that's fairly straightforward—nutrient-dense plant foods with low calories.

Dr. John McDougall's approach is not that different but with a few small twists. He suggests whole grains, starchy vegetables, colored vegetables, potatoes, and limited fruits. A similar approach is used by Dr. Michael Klaper. Professor Colin Campbell is also on board with complete avoidance of animal-sourced foods and advocates what he labels a whole-food plant-based diet (WFPB). Dr. Caldwell Esselstyn agrees with Campbell that the WFPB diet, with no added oils, is the best to prevent all non-communicable disease (NCDs) and holds the greatest promise for healing these ailments. It is clear to see where the major areas of agreement lie.

THE CRITERIA FOR A HEALTHY DIET

There are five criteria that can guide us in creating a healthy diet. These criteria are consistent with a vision of creating the healthiest human ecology possible. If we refer back to the rules of ecology, the first rule is that "everything is connected." This rule is not abstract; it is absolute and unchangeable.

It is not a coincidence that foods that promote personal health also have economic, social, environmental, and even psychological advantages. When we view these factors as "side benefits," we miss the point. When personal action is a reflection of natural justice, a state of biological integrity is achieved. This is the condition we call health. We like to focus our attention on the minutiae, but that is often not helpful.

The lack of compassion for life other than our own, the lack of appreciation for nature, the fear of change, and the frantic searches for instant gratification that characterize our society are woven into our food choices. Unravelling them is fundamental to creating a human ecology that allows us to reach our full potential.

When the following five principles are adhered to we are making healthy choices—further apart they are, the unhealthier the choices are.

1. *Nutritional Essentials:* It is well established what factors are essential for good nutrition. The primary features of water, carbohydrates, protein, fats, minerals, and vitamins are fairly well understood. The

only question is where we source them and in what quantities they should be in the diet. A healthy diet contains all the essential nutrients in combination to produce health and reduce sickness. This is the priority—create health. You will find a listing of these essentials in Chapter 13 .

2. *Social Justice:* There is an important social element to the foods we eat. The feeding of the family, society, nation, and the world should be of great concern to us all. Food justice means that the resources of good nutrition are available to all. It is important that food resources are available to everyone. The present food system is aimed at feeding only the affluent countries and creating profit for multi-national corporations. Food justice also means that the food we eat is not produced through the exploitation of others.

3. *Environmental Sustainability:* There is adequate information available as to the environmental impact of various foods. Factors such as water use and contamination, efficient land use, the demands of crops and animals for land clearing, soil erosion, and greenhouse gas emissions are some of these concerns. It would be suicidal to create a diet that killed the very source of our life.

4. *Ecological Integrity:* Moving toward a more productive dynamic with our environment can be greatly helped by introducing regional and seasonal consumption. Awareness of natural cycles and the local environment can greatly enhance the acceptance of a simpler, more nourishing food chain. This process is further promoted by learning life skills, such as cooking and home gardening.

5. *Ethical Clarity:* Changing the nutrition paradigm will mean that individuals will have to exhibit clarity in their decision-making process and be accountable for their food habits. The new approach to nutrition must be soundly based on honoring all life and the clear intention to avoid harm and exploitation to all animals, human and nonhuman alike.

These principles gain credence when communicated with kindness and the desire to make nutrition part of a progressive way of living that is based on personal, social, and environmental justice.

THE NUTRITIONAL ESSENTIALS

There is a general agreement that the modern diet—heavily dependent on animal fats, sugar, chemical additives, and trans fats—is killing us. Those populations that consume this diet consistently present the highest rates of NCDs. This has been shown in epidemiological studies since the 1950s and confirmed consistently by numerous studies.

Against these studies, there has been a recent curious upswing in contradictory reports that claim that these decades of study are incorrect and that "reasonable amounts" of saturated fats and even trans fats are acceptable. All the fuss was caused by a study that the Harvard School of Public Health labelled "seriously misleading." One of the reports in a popular medical site listed the lead author as "previously awarded a Dairy Innovation Australia grant, separate to this project."

These reports grab the attention of the popular press but never expose their bias. Even "science magazines" and science reporters love a controversy. Mark Bittman (mentioned earlier in Chapter Eleven) headlined an article joyfully entitled "Butter Is Back!" Can you imagine the joy?

The anomalies that can be found in the world populations are often tribal people or those living in unique social or environmental niches where they have adapted over many generations. These adaptations may include actions as diverse as cultural structures against eating too much, extremes of climate, poor soil, religious influences, or type of physical activity. Any of these factors can be important for creating results vastly different from the bulk of humanity. These reports are similar to the stories I often hear of the great-uncle that eats lard and smokes a pack of cigarettes a day but lives to be a lively ninety-two. It's an interesting story but meaningless in the big picture.

Stories of Maasai warriors, people living in deep jungles, or native Inuit people are interesting, but they are anomalies. They are not particularly germane to the discussion of a healthy diet in today's world and are quite often misleading. If our diet cannot feed everyone, there is a serious disconnect in our thinking.

The same is true of our real or imagined ancestors following the "traditional diet." The physical and social environment we live in has changed dramatically in the last century—even in the past fifty years. And it will keep on changing. It is the reality of the present, not the past, that we must make balance with. It is the present that produces the challenges to our health. Tradition is interesting and often instructive, but it is not always a sensible guideline for the future.

Diet as Therapy

We might also look at the difference between the therapeutic effects of diet as compared with maintenance. Much of what is written about diet is based on small studies using people who volunteer or individuals who follow a particular diet, get great results, and write a book. This is certainly interesting information, but we often have no way of assessing these stories. Is it possible that someone can get great results with a health issue (medically confirmed results) from doing something that is not really the best route for others, even if it works for some of them too? The answer is yes.

Health is about creating balance. If your life is extremely unbalanced and you make a drastic change, it will bring results. Sometimes the results are very beneficial. I have known clients or students who have recovered from a variety of illnesses by quitting their job, getting a divorce, moving house, or eating only one food for weeks on end. Life is mysterious sometimes. When they return to their doctors, they may be told that the results are "spontaneous remission" or incorrect diagnosis or an act of God. That does not mean that eating only avocado and coconut smoothies is the best path for everyone with that problem or that you could or should follow that program for the rest of your life.

In the macrobiotic community during the 1960s and '70s, there were many hundreds of people who changed to a particular diet and achieved better health. They were transitioning from an American diet. Some of them continued eating a more restrictive diet because of the results. Several problems emerged over time because they were using a diet that was designed for a specific purpose, and that purpose had changed.

Importance of Diversity

Diversity is important. If any diet is too restrictive, it becomes counterproductive. You cannot micromanage your nutrition. We all need a variety of taste and texture in food since food is a major form of pleasure.

We need to ask if a diet that is focused on reducing weight or lowering cholesterol or stabilizing blood sugar levels is essential for a healthy life once the target is achieved. I am not talking about returning to a diet that may have been the cause of the problem; I am addressing adjustment.

One of the things noticed by macrobiotic practitioners was that a no-oil or a very low-oil diet was very helpful in shrinking cancer tumors and reducing cholesterol levels but was often difficult to sustain. Part of the problem was in achieving a variety of textures and mouth feel without oil. By the mid-1980s, it was standard advice to prohibit all oil for the best results.

It is interesting that it is the oil controversy that separates most of the abovementioned doctors and professionals. There is no question that the reduction of oil provides the best results in reversing all the NCDs. The question for me is what next? The controversy will probably continue since everyone loves the micro issues.

The essentials of carbohydrates, proteins, fats, minerals, and vitamins are easily available in a diet comprised of grains, beans, vegetables, seeds, nuts, and fruits. The addition of some fermented foods (both vegetables and soy products) and small amounts of sea vegetables form the basis of a macrobiotic human ecology diet.

SOCIAL JUSTICE

Food has always been a shared resource. Archaeologists working in Israel at the Qesem Cave site have unearthed what they have identified as the first shared hearth where food was cooked and used for communal food preparation and sharing. The earliest findings are dated some three hundred thousand years ago.

Both hunter-gatherers and agriculturalists lived in cultures where food was acknowledged as a simple right. Food captured or grown was always made available to everyone in the tribe or village. It has always been part of our humanity to offer food to those in need. Pearl Buck, an American Nobel Prize winning author, stated:

Food for all is a necessity. Food should not be a merchandise, to be bought and sold as jewels are bought and sold by those who have the money to buy. Food is a human necessity—like water and air, it should be available.

Every culture has its own food rituals. Any world traveller can tell you that eating a meal in Italy is a different experience from dining in India. It's not simply the food—it is the cultural attitude about food and how it is shared. The foods used, the etiquette, and the conversations are all woven into the fabric of daily life.

Food has always been a reflection of the environment and seasonal change. The fatty foods and alcohol in deep winter festivals when dark months reach their nadir and the days start to lengthen are an example of this, as well as the spring festivals when fertility is celebrated. These festivals always featured sharing food and were part of the biological shift required to create balance.

One of the concepts that has been common within macrobiotic thinking is the fact that sharing food is a way of creating similar blood quality. It is seen as part of the binding force of family. What are the implications of this when most food is manufactured outside the home and individuals within a single family eat extremely diverse diets? One in four Americans eats at least one fast-food meal every single day. In 2007, 37.4 percent of food eaten away from home was purchased from limited-service restaurants, such as fast-food outlets. One effect of this fracture in family eating has been studied fairly extensively.

Children and the Family Meal

Using data from nearly three-quarters of the world's countries, an analysis by the Organization for Economic Cooperation and Development (OECD) found that students who do not regularly eat with their parents are significantly more likely to be truant at school. The average truancy rate in the two weeks before the Program for International Student Assessment (PISA)—a test administered to fifteen-year-olds by the OECD and used in the analysis as a measure for absenteeism—was about 15 percent throughout the world on average, but it was nearly 30 percent when pupils reported they didn't often share meals with their families.

Those students who did not eat dinner with parents were 40 percent more likely to be overweight compared to those who do. Children who do eat dinner with their parents five or more days a week have less trouble with drugs and alcohol, eat healthier, show better academic performance, and report being closer with their parents than children who eat dinner with their parents less often.

These studies do not give tremendous insight into the social and economic conditions that might make family meals difficult. One glaring fact is that the focus in many of them is obesity and not on the childhood onset of diabetes, cancers, and the beginnings of heart disease that are the real issue. Society at large and the less well-off in particular are being led away from health by commercial interests. No matter how many well-meaning after-school exercise programs begin, the tidal surge of poor health among the poor and particularly the poor urban youth will continue.

The nutritional nightmare that started in America has now spread around the world through the power of nutritional colonialism. Nutritional epidemiologist Youfa Wang from Johns Hopkins Bloomberg School of Public Health studied the dramatic rise in obesity among children in sixty-seven countries around the world. Childhood obesity in China was of particular interest since it has risen faster than any other nation over the past few years.

As part of the study, he tracked the rise of Kentucky Fried Chicken restaurants in China for over two and a half decades. In 1987, the first franchise set out its shingle; by 2010, 3,700 were in business, concentrated primarily on the urban east coast, where obesity rates are the highest. This link between childhood obesity and junk food is no longer limited to wealthy nations. Mexico, India, and Brazil have joined America, Canada, and Australia in the race to undermine the health of the next generation. Wang and his colleagues found that children had become heavier in the sixty-seven countries studied and that the rise was attributed to fast-food consumption.

Much is made of the issue of feeding the world; it is an important issue, but only if we ask what we feed the world with. Food justice is essential, and the availability of healthy food should be a priority in all countries. There is little relationship between the volume of food eaten and malnutrition. There are many people, both young and old, that are starving from lack of basic nutrition and eating the calorically dense and nutrient-poor diets sold at fast-food outlets and supermarkets. Our participation in maintaining the power of an unhealthy food industry is going to be reflected in the health of the next generation; they will not thank us.

Social justice in nutrition also needs to be concerned with how our choices affect those invisible people who grow or process our food—food slavery. I focused on this issue in Chapter Ten, "Collateral Damage." We need to be aware of the damage done to those who produce our food. This is not only about those in Africa, South America, or Asia—but those at home. This means finding out about where our food comes from and doing research into the working conditions and payment to those who grow, process, and pack our food.

ENVIRONMENTAL SUSTAINABILITY

In 1895, a Swedish scientist by the name of Svante Arrhenius approached the question of potential atmospheric warming due to the presence of heat-absorbing gases. It was a hobby for this Nobel Prize winner. His predictions, made with pen and paper, were nearly spot-on. Arrhenius was unambiguous regarding the reasons the climate would get warmer. The increases in carbon dioxide were due to the increased human activities of combustion processes and burning coal. He was not concerned with this warming and felt that it might even be sort of nice if the weather became warmer (remember he lived in Sweden). Now we know better.

So 120 years later, we are still debating the issue in the face of mounting evidence that climate change is real and dangerous to all life on the planet. Over 97 percent of all scientific papers on the science of climate confirm that the changes in the atmosphere are primarily driven by human activity and that they are a threat to human society. The effect of continuing with the activities producing climate change will contribute to a constellation of impacts. There will be more droughts and heat waves (contributing to increased wildfires) and stronger hurricanes and increased flooding in some areas due to changes in the weather patterns.

Many plant and animal species are threatened as habitats change. These changes affect both land and sea life, leading to increased extinction of many species. There will be a rise in sea levels even if swift action is taken. One of the greatest natural factors to mitigate this warming trend and reduce atmospheric CO_2 would be forests. The positive influence of forestland is diminished mostly by the clearing of land to grow feed for animals. This lessens the number of trees. In addition, dying trees release held CO_2, further complicating the problem.

When we look at the effect of our food choices on climate change, the solution is obvious. Meat and all forms of animal agriculture are the most significant direct contributor to the problem. Livestock production accounts for up to 70 percent of all agricultural land use and 30 percent of the land surface of the planet. According to the United Nations, livestock contributes 18 percent of greenhouse gases and is a major contributor to both land and water degradation. The bottom line is that if you care about saving the environment and still have meat, fish, dairy, or eggs on the menu, you need to think again.

Using animals as a food source is short-sighted in terms of the environment, but so is eating most of the food produced by the international food giants. Agribusiness is a major polluter to both living and non-living systems in the environment. Those abiotic (non-living) factors include damage to soil through erosion, waste and pollution of groundwater, rivers, and lakes, and leaching of minerals from the soil.

Aside from increased sedimentation in rivers, the intensive use of herbicides and pesticides kill off not only the insects harmful to crops but also those that are beneficial, such as pollinators. The chemicals, along with artificial fertilizers, leach into groundwater and rivers, making their way to the oceans where they turn large swaths of sea into "dead zones."

The production of our food is killing the environment that produces the foods we are living on. The same chemicals that poison the insects, the river life, and the microorganisms in the soil poison us as well. Why would we want to feed toxic food to ourselves and our children? Organic, local, and seasonal food is a major step toward a deeper personal ecology and improved health.

ECOLOGICAL INTEGRITY

We are a product of our environment. The natural tendency of our body is to bring itself into alignment with the soil, climate, season, natural vegetation, and water that surrounds us. As much as possible, we would be wise to align ourselves to the natural rhythms and effects of our habitat. For some people, this may be difficult due to urban life, but it is not impossible. Following a few simple rules is helpful.

Consuming food in season is a great place to start. You will feel the difference. Buying locally grown foods is an advantage not only to the individual but in supporting local farmers and increasing their share of the market. Small farms produce the bulk of the world's food. It is easier for small farmers to grow organically, and many do. Supporting local and regional farms is a good way to begin creating food security and eating food that reflects our natural habitat.

This process involves renewing simple life skills. Among the most important of these skills is the cooking and home processing of our food. Learning a variety of simple cooking methods is not difficult. It requires a little time, but this is not haute cuisine—it is folk cooking. It can reflect the culture of any country. It can be as delicious, artistic, and as imaginative as you want, but the basics are simple, tasty, hearty, and healthy.

Home food processing also includes home fermentation and sprouting. Sauerkraut, pickles, vegan kimchi, and pressed salads are very easy to produce and use throughout the year. Sourdough bread is also in this category. These foods all enroll the service of local yeasts and bacteria in the air to enhance the quality of the final product.

Growing our own food, wherever possible, is a great way to establish bio integrity. Having our own garden or sharing garden space with others allows us to participate in the cycle of the seasons—to understand the way our food is grown and to better form the link between ourselves and nature. All these simple acts are intended to take back the relationship between what we eat and where we live. They are undertakings that bring increased control over our lives and to better exercise control over our collective health and well-being.

ETHICAL CLARITY

The issue of food ethics is a minefield of social conflict. Those of us who have been raised in liberal democratic societies expect a high degree of personal freedom and expect that freedom as an "inalienable" right. We feel entitled to make certain life choices without interference from the State. This is, of course, not the case. We are nations of laws.

If I am angry at my neighbor, I will be taken to court and punished if I attack him or destroy his property. If I have a prejudice against another race or religion, I may be censured if I translate that prejudice into violent or demeaning speech or actions. We refine these laws over time to adapt to increased knowledge or social change. Because of the cultural, emotional, and sensorial role that food plays in our lives, we have placed it off-limits.

If a food product contains enough poison or contamination to kill, we are outraged and demand it be removed—but only if the effect is swift and dramatic. If there are ingredients that slowly erode our health, we feel no need to act quickly but would rather wait and see if our suspicions are valid. This is especially true if the item in question is tasty, comforting to us, believed to be traditional or thought to contain magical ingredients.

The attack on the Twin Towers on September 11, 2001 killed 2,996 people and injured 6,000 others. The monetary cost of the damage was estimated at $10 billion. The response to the attack was a war that, as of this writing, cost in excess of $5 trillion. The number of coalition troops killed in Iraq alone was put at 4,424 and almost as many wounded. According to Iraq Body Count, an independent US/UK project, the lowest estimated counts of civilians killed was between 155,923 to 174,355. This is an extremely shallow picture of the human misery of these events and does not mention the impact on children without parents, families displaced, or men and women who live with devastating disability. What would it be like if we applied the same commitment to products that kill an excess of those numbers?

We all feel the grief and sadness, perhaps even anger at this senseless destruction. Nations become irate when their citizens are killed by a foreign power, and they lash out. They will spend a treasure and kill the innocent to avenge the crime. When the deaths are caused by the function of respected business, it seems a different rule of law applies.

A study by researchers at MIT found that 200,000 deaths each year were linked to air pollution. We know that the automobile and power companies are responsible for the largest contribution to this problem. Cigarette smoke causes 480,000 deaths annually in the USA and 6 million deaths worldwide. We know who makes them. In 2002, the US surgeon general, David Satcher, issued a "call to action" in response to the fact that 300,000 deaths each year were related to obesity—the main cause being fast food. We know who makes it.

PRINCIPLES INTO PRACTICE

If you agree with the criteria for good nutrition I have been presenting above there is only one thing left to do – start applying them in your daily life. You may look at my recommendations and say, "This is going to be difficult." My answer is always the same—"If you believe that it will be." It may be comforting to know that most folks settle into a new rhythm of healthy stress-free living by simply following these simple guidelines.

Know What You Want

You may be making changes in your food choices for your health or the animals or the environment (maybe all three) but be clear on your reasons. Align your mind and your emotions behind your vision. Some people take only a few days to adjust to a new diet, some a few weeks. It is a learning process; simply keep focused on your goals. Expect it to be easy and it will be.

Physical Adaptions

Some people expect that there will be a negative reaction when they cut out familiar foods; that is seldom the case. Stopping the use of strong stressors, such as coffee or cigarettes, can produce headaches on occasion as "withdrawal symptoms," but that is rare. The cells of the body are under constant replacement, some on a daily basis, some weekly or monthly; you are nourishing new growth. Let your body do what it is designed to do. Give your body the right tools and it knows how to build health.

Fast or Slow

Taking baby steps is not the best way to reach a destination. You want to be able to experience the full benefit of your actions and create a contrast. Those who do the "meatless Monday" or "flexarian" approach usually stick right there. It is easy to feel like we made progress and be satisfied. I always want more for my readers; I want them to have the full experience.

Read Labels

Creating a healthy and ethical diet means taking back control of your health and your kitchen. The very same mentality that created the crisis in food production is now moving into the "natural," "plant based," and "vegan" food arena. As an intelligent consumer you will read labels carefully and not buy into the new junk food in the market place. Buy simple whole foods in their natural state wherever possible and organic whenever you can.

Use Skill Power Not Willpower

Learn to cook! You don't need to be a polished chef to make simple tasty meals. Find a range of recipes that satisfy your taste-buds and focus on them to begin with. You can expand your variety slowly. There are plenty of cookbooks available. On my website you can get downloads of free recipes. There is nothing like tasty food to keep you on track.

Plan to Win

If you have it in your kitchen you will eat it. If you can, clean out your cupboard, get rid of all the junk. You can give it to friends (or enemies). That half gallon of Hagen Daz in the fridge will be eaten by you in a moment of weakness. Stock up on healthy food, and that's what you will eat. This doesn't mean "healthy junk." Read labels, there are many products that claim to be healthy that aren't—don't fall for it.

Stay Positive

Some of the biggest problems that some people face when changing their food choices is not the food but the people around them. Friends, family, and even casual acquaintances turn out to be nutritional experts.

Don't be defensive, stick with what you know and refer people to do some reading. There are tons of references at the end of the book, there is no reason for you to get into arguments. On the other hand...

Education

...education is a good idea. Check out the references, read the books of those doctors and nutritionists I have referred to, but keep it simple. You don't need to be a professional to eat well. Sometimes people get drowned with all the information. Trust your experience. Stick with the guidelines I have presented and give yourself time.

Have Fun

This is not a task; it is an honor to eat in a way that produces health for both humans and non-humans. With health comes a simplicity of life and a vitality to do whatever it is you want. This is not about guilt and grief; it is about celebrating life.

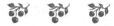

We are faced with a truly unique challenge. It is one that human life has never experienced before and if not resolved well may be the deciding factor in the human experiment. A sense of urgency is surely needed. That urgency requires massive education that avoids the pitfalls of panicking or patronising. The answer is clear values that can resonate with the individual desire for health and satisfying food. We can expect no help from the food industry and only limited assistance from organized medicine.

The sea changes in food choices are seen primarily as a market opportunity by "Big Food." It is easy to change formulas to conform to shifts in the market. The problem is that if the request is always to "leave something out" it creates new problems. A new food ethic that has positive demands for food content is more powerful.

If the consumer demands whole-foods, unadulterated and grown according to free-trade and organic standards, the message is clear. If the request is simply to reduce or eliminate oils, gluten, sugar or any of a long list of ingredients, it opens the door for suspect replacements. Industry will always find a way to cut corners to generate more profit. The best future is achieved by using whole natural foods and making the home kitchen the center of food processing.

Human nutritional needs are simple and do not require a great deal of analysis. It is not helpful to attempt to micro-manage personal nutritional needs. The listing of foods in the previous two chapters, with proper diversity is sufficient in most cases. I always suggest that clients eat the diet as described in Chapter Thirteen for two to four weeks and see how they feel. I have never had anyone say they didn't feel better. That does not mean that diet is a panacea—much goes into good health, but a healthy diet is always required.

$\mathcal{C}$onclusion

When I was a child in California we would go camping every summer. We would set up our campsite in the Sierra Nevada Mountains and spend a week or two walking, fishing, or swimming in the rivers or lakes. There was abundant wildlife in the forest if you were willing to sit quiet and wait. You could see fish swimming in the streams and you could drink out of any of the big rivers. All that has changed. The forest floor is littered with trash, huge swaths of land have been logged, and rivers are fished out and polluted. The marks of humankind dominate the landscape.

Weekly, if not daily, we hear that the world is in danger. It is widely accepted that human activity is the source of the threat. We are consigning ourselves and future generations to a world where those systems that give us life and pleasure will be harmed beyond repair. The world is on fire and most wait to see if some political, scientific hero or intervention from a benevolent god will solve the problem—it is a futile and dangerous wait. Only a transformation of the heart and mind can transform this impending tragedy into the greatest revolution in human cultural history. It is up to us.

Over the course of these pages I have presented what I feel is the most important part of this revolution. It is so simple that it is easily set aside as trivial or a fad and not bold enough to match the magnitude of the problem. After all, the issue involves governments, big business, and social habit. It is in its simplicity that lays its greatest power.

There is no act too small, no act too bold. The history of social change is the history of millions of actions, small and large, coming

274

together at critical points to create a power that governments cannot suppress.

—Howard Zinn, historian

HEART AND MIND, BODY AND SOUL

Changing our food choices is an act of Deep Ecology. It is a practical demonstration of our personal awareness of our link to nature. This automatically places us outside the social environment we live in; it encourages us to pay attention. It is an act of rebellion against the consumption of toxic foods built on social injustice, ecological damage, and the killing of sentient life. It is an escape from the most prevalent aspect of consumerism. It is difficult to imagine a single act that has so many positive repercussions to our physical, social, and psychological well-being.

As we move into an era where our young are developing the diseases of the old, where behavioral problems continue to rise, and our health systems teeter on the edge of failure, we should be worried. That is seemingly not the case. We are held in place by deep-seated emotional attachments and outdated traditions.

Imagine the benefit of preventing 50 percent of all heart disease, reducing cancers by 30 percent, or reversing 80 percent of all type two diabetes. Think of the impact on our overworked hospitals, doctors, and nurses. I believe that the figures above are conservative. Achieving them would require no new drugs, no improved technologies, and no extensive training of professionals. What it will require is a new vision of health and healing as well as a stronger commitment to real rather than superficial change.

What should draw our interest is the resistance to significant food reforms, particularly where the end of animal use is part of the plan. This will come regardless of our resistance; we need to set the foundation for a healthy transition. It is telling that no major environmental organization suggests veganism as a viable act to slow and even reverse climate change. This is true even though the science is very clear; it is the most significant thing individuals can do to create change. The suggestions to "reduce" consumption are baffling.

We are encouraged instead to cut down on air travel, use of cars, or products shipped long distance even though simply avoiding all animal sourced foods far out-strips the impact of all these together. Even so-called "animal welfare" groups, who depend on donations to exist, will not make a firm statement against the killing. They focus on the comfort level of the animals prior to slaughter. This position basically says that it is the comfort level before the killing that is the problem, not the killing.

One of the clear lessons we can learn from our present dilemma is that nutrition, health, ecological concerns, and compassion for non-human life are all intimately linked. Until we approach human activities with a clear ethic regarding long term outcome we are doomed to flounder from the effects of simplistic solutions. The Iroquois Council of tribal affairs encouraged leaders to consider the impact of decisions for seven generations. Try and imagine what today's leaders would decide if that system had the force of law. In today's rush for the quick fix they would be paralyzed, but it must be done. It is a challenge to us all.

The food industry and the damage it does from farm to factory to table will only change through consumer demands. These demands should not be for "vegan" or "healthy" replacements for familiar junk food. Our demands should be for food that is organically grown and free of chemicals; it needs to be whole food and not processed quick fixes. The more we move our attention back into the kitchen, the more control we have over our health and our relationship to the environment. This in no way needs to inhibit any other social actions we wish to take or other environmental causes we want to pursue, but it is fundamental.

My wife Marlene and I have 90 years of experience between us in the field of natural health care. Our website, www.macrovegan.org is a good source of information for putting the ideas in this book into practice. The fact that you are reading this conclusion is a first step to understand the problems and what each of us can do. The next steps you take, however, are the crucial ones. What can you do on a personal level to live a more healthful existence and, in turn, spread the word to others? Just know that we are here to support your shift to eating a diet that is healthy and causes no harm; we welcome your questions. After all if we don't take care of our body and our planet, where are we going to live?

References

Chapter 1

Accum, F. *A Treatise on Adulterations of Food and Culinary Poisons*. London: Longman, 1820.

Blumenthal, D., Campbell, E.G., Causino, N., Louis, K.S. "Participation of life-science faculty in research relationships with industry." *N Engl J Med* 1996 Dec 5; 335(23):1734–9.

Blythman, J. *Swallow This: Serving Up the Food Industry's Darkest Secrets*. London: 4th Estate, 1988.

Food Ingredient Facts. https://www.foodingredientfacts.org.

FoodPrint. https://foodprint.org

GAO. "FDA Should Strengthen Its Oversight of Food Ingredients Determined to Be Generally Recognized as Safe (GRAS)." GAO-10-246: Published: Feb 3, 2010. Publicly Released: Mar 5, 2010. 10.1016/j.jada.2010.07.010.

Institute of Medicine. *Dietary Reference Intakes for Energy, Carbohydrate, Fiber, Fat, Fatty Acids, Cholesterol, Protein, and Amino Acids*. Washington, DC: the National Academies Press, 2005. https://doi.org/10.17226/10490.

Lau, K., McLean, W.G., Williams, D.P., Howard, C.V. "Synergistic interactions between commonly used food additives in a developmental neurotoxicity test." *Toxicology Science* 2006 Mar; 90(1):178–87.

Lenard I Lesser, Cara B. Ebbeling, Merrill Goozner, David Wypij, and David S Ludwig. Martijn Katan, Academic Editor. "Relationship between Funding Source and Conclusion among Nutrition-Related Scientific Articles." *PLoS Med*. 2007 Jan; 4(1): e5.

Life. March 6, 1970. Page 38.

McDonald's Nutrition Calculator. http://nutrition.mcdonalds.com/getnutrition/ingredientslist.pdf.

OECD (2011), *Society at a Glance 2011 - OECD Social Indicators* (www.oecd.org/social/societyataglance2011.htm)

Poti, J.M., Popkin, B.M. "Trends in Energy Intake among US Children by Eating Location and Food Source, 1977–2006." *J Am Diet Assoc.* 2011; 111:1, 156–1,164.

Reedy, J., Krebs-Smith, S. "Dietary Sources of Energy, Solid Fats, and Added Sugars among Children and Adolescents in the United States." *J Am Diet Assoc.* 2010; 110:1477–1484. doi:

Subway Nutrition. https://www.subway.com/en-US/MenuNutrition/Nutrition/WhatsInOurFood.

Chapter 2

Armstrong, B., Doll, R. "Environmental factors and cancer incidence and mortality in different countries, with special reference to dietary practices." *Int J Cancer* 1975 Apr 15; 15(4): 617–631.

Barnard, Neal. Physicians Committee for Responsible Medicine, Understanding Health, December, 1999. www.pcrm.org/health-topics/healthy-bones.

Braga, D.P., Halpern, G., Figueira Rde, C., Setti, A.S., Iaconelli, A Jr., Borges, E Jr. "Food intake and social habits in male patients and its relationship to intracytoplasmic sperm injection outcomes." *Fertil Steril.* 2012 Jan; 97(1): 53–59.

Cadogan, J., Eastell, R., Jones, N., Barker, M.E. "Milk intake and bone mineral acquisition in adolescent girls: randomized, controlled intervention trial." *BMJ* 1997; 315:1255–69.

Carroll, K.K., Braden, L.M. "Dietary fat and mammary carcinogenesis." *Nutrition and Cancer* 1985; 6:254–259.

Chan, J.M., Stampfer, M.J., Giovannucci, E., et al. "Plasma insulin-like growth factor-1 and prostate cancer risk: a prospective study." *Science* 1998; 279:563–5.

Chavarro, J.E., Rich-Edwards, J.W., Rosner, B.A., et al. "Protein intake and ovulatory infertility." *Am J Obstet Gynecol.* 2008; 198:210.e1–210.e7.

Feskanich, D., Willett, W.C., and Colditz, G.A. "Calcium, vitamin D, milk consumption, and hip fractures: a prospective study among postmenopausal women." *American Journal of Clinical Nutrition* 2003 Feb; 77(2); 504–11.

Feskanich, D., Willett, W.C., Colditz, G.A. "Calcium, vitamin D, milk consumption, and hip fractures: a prospective study among postmenopausal women." *Am J Clin Nutr.* 2003; 77:504–511.

Giovannucci, E., Rimm, E.B., Colditz, G.A., Stampfer, M.J., Ascherio, A., Chute, C.C., Willett, W.C. "A prospective study of dietary fat and risk of prostate cancer." *J Natl Cancer Inst.* 1993; 85(19):1,571–1,579.

Hardy, K., Buckley, S., Collins, M.J., et al. "Neanderthal medics? Evidence for food, cooking, and medicinal plants entrapped in dental calculus." *Naturwissenschaften* August 2012; Volume 99, Issue 8, pp. 617–626.

Huang, T., Xu, M., Lee, A., Cho, S., Qi, L. "Consumption of whole grains and cereal fiber and total and cause-specific mortality: prospective analysis of 367,442 individuals." *BMC Medicine* 2015 Mar 24; 13:59.

Isaacs, E.B., Fischl, B.R., Quin, B.T., et al. "Impact of breast milk on IQ, brain size, and white matter development." *Pediatr Res.* 2010 Apr; 67(4): 357–362.

Johns Hopkins Medicine. *Diabetes Education #15.* "No More Carb Confusion." www.hopkinsmedicine.org/gim/core_resources/patient%20handouts/handouts_may_2012/no%20more%20carb%20confusion.pdf.

Journal of Archaeological Science November 1995; Volume 22, Issue 6.

Journal of the American Dietetic Association July 2009.

Kolonel, L.N. "Nutrition and prostate cancer." *Cancer Causes Control* 1996 Jan; 7(1); 83–94.

Lanou, A.J., Berkow, S.E., Barnard, N.D. "Calcium, dairy products, and bone health in children and young adults: a reevaluation of the evidence." *Pediatrics* 2005; 115:736–743.

Oldways Whole Grain Council. "Existing Standards for Whole Grains." http://wholegrainscouncil.org/whole-grains-101/existing-standards-for-whole-grains.

Robbana-Barnat, S., Rabache, M., Rialland, E., Fradin, J. "Heterocyclic amines: occurrence and prevention in cooked food." *Environ Health Perspect.* 1996; 104:280–288.

Ruxton, C.H., Gardner, E.J., McNulty, H.M. "Is Sugar Consumption Detrimental to Health? A Review of Evidence" 1995–2006." *Critical Reviews in Food Science and Nutrition* Jan; 50(1):1–19.

Skog, K.I., Johansson, M.A.E., Jagerstad, M.I. Carcinogenic heterocyclic amines in model systems and cooked foods: a review on formation, occurrence, and intake. *Food and Chem Toxicol.* 1998 Sep–Oct; 36(9–10):879–896.

Smith, Roff. "Oldest Known Hearth Found in Israel Cave." *National Geographic* January 29, 2014. https://news.nationalgeographic.com/news/2014/01/140129-oldest-hearth-israel-cave-new-human-species-discovery-archaeology-science.

Taubes, G., Kearns Couzens, C. *Mother Jones* November/December 2012 Issue.

USDA's Economic Research Service, Year 2000. "Americans' Whole-Grain Consumption Below Guidelines." www.ers.usda.gov/amber-waves/2005/april/americans-whole-grain-consumption-below-guidelines.

Chapter 3

Bailer, J. Annual Meeting of the American Association for the Advancement of Science in May 1985.

Binder, Leah. "Stunning News on Preventable Deaths in Hospitals." *Forbes* Sep. 23, 2013. https://www.forbes.com/sites/leahbinder/2013/09/23/stunning-news-on-preventable-deaths-in-hospitals/#69886ee64f69.

Blaser, M.J., Falkow, S. "What are the consequences of the disappearing human microbiota?" *Nat Rev Microbiol.* 2009 Dec; 7(12):887–94.

Centers for Disease Control and Prevention. *Antibiotic Resistance in the United States, 2013.* https://www.cdc.gov/drugresistance/pdf/ar-threats-2013-508.pdf

Centers for Disease Control and Prevention. National Diabetes Statistics Report, 2014. https://www.cdc.gov/diabetes/pdfs/data/2014-report-estimates-of-diabetes-and-its-burden-in-the-united-states.pdf.

Dinse, G.E., Umbach, D.M., Sasco, A.J., et al. "Unexplained increases in cancer incidence in the United States from 1975 to 1994." *Annual Review of Public Health* 1999; 20:173–209.

Epstein, H. "Flu Warning: Beware the Drug Companies." The *New York Review of Books* May 12, 2011.

Ferlay, J., Soerjomataram, I., et al. "Cancer incidence and mortality worldwide: sources, methods and major patterns in GLOBOCAN 2012." *Int J Cancer* 2015 Mar 1; 136(5):E359-86.

Feskanich D, Willett WC, and Colditz, GA. "Calcium, vitamin D, milk consumption, and hip fractures: a prospective study among postmenopausal women." *American Journal of Clinical Nutrition* 2003 Feb; 77(2):504–11.

Go, A.S., Mozaffarian, D., Roger, V.L., Benjamin, E.J., Berry, J.D., Blaha, M.J., et al. "Heart disease and stroke statistics—2014 update: a report from the American Heart Association." *Circulation* 2014 Jan 21; 129(3):e28–e292.

Heidenreich, P.A., Trogdon, J.G., Khavjou, O.A., et al. "Forecasting the future of cardiovascular disease in the United States: a policy statement from the American Heart Association." *Circulation* 2011 Mar 1; 123(8):933–44.

Lim, E.L., Hollingsworth, K.G., Aribasala, B.S., et al. "Reversal of type 2 diabetes: normalisation of beta cell function in association with decreased pancreas and liver triacylglycerol." *Diabetologia* 2011 Oct; 54(10):2506–14.

Mayo Clinic, Drugs and Supplements, Armodafinil. www.mayoclinic.org/drugs-supplements/armodafinil-oral-route/side-effects/drg-20071125.

Mendelsohn, Robert S. *Confessions of a Medical Heretic.* Chicago, IL: Contemporary Books, 1979.

Murphy, S.L., Xu, J.Q., Kochanek, K.D. "Deaths: Final data for 2010." *Natl Vital Stat Rep* 2013 May 8; 61(4):1–117.

Knapton, S. "'Soft touch' doctors should be disciplined for over-prescribing antibiotics." The *Telegraph* 18 Aug 2015. www.telegraph.co.uk/news/science/science-news/11808015/Soft-touch-doctors-should-be-disciplined-for-over-prescribing-antibiotics.html.

OECD (2013), Health at a Glance 2013: OECD Indicators, OECD Publishing. http://dx.doi.org/10.1787/health_glance-2013-en.

Ruesch, H. *Naked Empress, or the Great Medical Fraud.* Massagno/Lugano, Switzerland: Civis Publicatrions, 1992.

Shaw, J.E., Sicree, R.A., Zimmet, P.Z. "Global estimates of the prevalence of diabetes for 2010 and 2030." *Diabetes Res Clin Pract.* 2010 Jan; 87(1):4–14.

World Health Organization. The *World Health Report 2000.* Geneva, Switzerland: World Health Organization, 2000.

Chapter 4

American Medical Association. "History of the Code." www.ama-assn.org/sites/ama-assn.org/files/corp/media-browser/public/ethics/ama-code-ethics-history.pdf.

Armstrong, B., Doll, R. "Environmental factors and cancer incidence and mortality in different countries, with special reference to dietary practices." *Int J Cancer* 1975 Apr 15; 15(4):617–31.

Beecher, Henry K. "Ethics and Clinical Research." *New England Journal of Medicine* 1966 June 16; 274(24): 1354–60.

Bush, Harold K. The *Letters of Mark Twain and Joseph Hopkins Twichell*. Athens, GA: University of Georgia Press, 2017.

Canadian Government Commission of Inquiry into the Non-Medical Use of Drugs. Ottawa, Canada: Information Canada, 1972, Crown Copyrights Reserved.

Ember, C.R., Ember, M., Eds. *Encyclopedia of Medical Anthropology: Health and Illness in the World's Cultures, Volume I: Topics, Volume II: Cultures*. New York: Springer, 2004.

Grimes, W. "Apr 24–30; How About Some Popcorn with Your Fat?" *New York Times* May 1, 1994.

Hammond, E.C., Horn, D. "The relationship between human smoking habits and death rates: a follow-up study of 187,766 men." *J Am Med Assoc*. 1954 Aug 7; 155(15):1316–28.

Herzberg, D. *Happy Pills in America*. Baltimore, MD: Johns Hopkins University Press, 2009.

Hirayama, T. "Epidemiology of breast cancer with special reference to the role of diet." *Prev Med*. 1978 Jun; 7(2):173-95.

Keys, A., Taylor, H.L., Blackburn, H., Brozek, J., Anderson, J.T., Simonson, E. "Coronary Heart Disease among Minnesota Business and Professional Men Followed Fifteen Years." *Circulation* 1963 Sep; 28:381-95.

Lappé, Frances Moore. *Diet for a Small Planet*. New York: Ballantine Books, 1971.

Lee, E.A., Angka, L., Rota, S.G., et al. "Targeting Mitochondria with Avocatin B Induces Selective Leukemia Cell Death." *Cancer Res* 2015 June 15; 75(12):2478–88.

Mahmood, S.S., Levy, D., Vasan, R.S., Wang, T.J. "The Framingham Heart Study and the epidemiology of cardiovascular disease: a historical perspective." *Lancet* 2014 Mar 15; 383(9921):999–1008.

Mayo Clinic Health Letter, June 2017. https://healthletter.mayoclinic.com/issues.

Nurses' Health Study. www.nurseshealthstudy.org.

Placek, P.J., Taffel, S.M. "Cesarean section delivery rates: United States, 1981." *Am J Public Health* 1983 August; 73(8):861–862.

Proctor, R.N. "The history of the discovery of the cigarette–lung cancer link: evidentiary traditions, corporate denial, global toll." *Tob Control* 2012 Mar; 21(2):87-91.

Robbins, J. *Diet for a New America*. Walpole, NH: Stillpoint Publishing, 1987.

Rosen G. "Benjamin Rush on health and the American revolution." *Am J Public Health* 1976 April; 66(4): 397–398.

Shurtleff, W., Aoyagi, A. The *History of Erewhon*. Lafayette, CA: Soyinfo Center, 2011.

Spock, B. The *Common Sense Book of Baby and Child Care*. New York: Duell, Sloan, and Pearce, 1946.

Stanford University Research into the Impact of Tobacco Advertising. "Cigarettes Advertising Themes." http://tobacco.stanford.edu/tobacco_main/main.php.

US Senate Select Committee on Nutrition and Human Needs. *Dietary Goals for the United States*. 2nd Edition. Washington, D.C.: US Govt. Print. Off., 1977.

Chapter 5

Angell, M. "Drug Companies and Doctors: A Story of Corruption." The *New York Review of Books* January 15, 2009. Vol. 56, no. 1.

Balkwill, F., Mantovani, A. "Inflammation and cancer: back to Virchow?" *Lancet* 2001 Feb 17; 357(9255):539-45.

Brill, S. "How much money is raised and spent on fighting cancer? *Reuters* September 9, 2014. www.reuters.com/article/idIN325322161920140909.

Calabresi, M. "Why America Can't Kick Its Painkiller Problem." *Time*. June 4, 2015. https://time.com/magazine/us/3908624/june-15th-2015-vol-185-no-22-u-s.

Centers for Disease Control and Prevention. "Chronic Disease Overview." Atlanta, GA: CDC, 2008.

Centers for Disease Control and Prevention. "Leading Causes of Death in America." Atlanta, GA: CDC, 2013.

Chen, J., Peto, R., Pan, W., et al. Eds. "Mortality, Biochemistry, Diet and Lifestyle in Rural China. Geographical Study of the characteristics of 69 Counties in mainland China and 16 Areas in Taiwan." *J Epidemiol Community Health* 2007 Mar; 61(3): 271.

Connor, S. "Glaxo chief: Our drugs do not work on most patients." *Independent* 8 December 2003. www.independent.co.uk/news/science/glaxo-chief-our-drugs-do-not-work-on-most-patients-5508670.html.

Corman, L.C. "Relationship between Nutrition, Infection, and Immunity." *Med Clin North Am*. 1985 May; 69(3):519-31.

Cuomo, M.I. *A World without Cancer*. New York: Rodale, 2012.

Dawber, T.R. The *Framingham Study: the Epidemiology of Atherosclerotic Disease*. Cambridge/London: Harvard University Press, 1980.

Endocrine Society and Hormone Foundation. The *Endocrine Society Weighs In: A Handbook on Obesity in America*. Chevy Chase, MD: Obesity in America, 2005.

Fanelli, D. "How many scientists fabricate and falsify research? A systematic review and meta-analysis of survey data." *PLoS One* 2009 May 29; 4(5):e5738.

Fang, F.C., Steen R.G., Casadevall, A. "Misconduct accounts for the majority of retracted scientific publications." *PNAS* October 16, 2012 109 (42) 17028-17033.

Faughnan, John G. "Alternative Medicine: A Critique from Scientific Medicine." www.faughnan.com.

Freedom of Information (FOI) request to the Scottish Ambulance Service, 2015.

Glade, M.J. "Food, nutrition, and the prevention of cancer: a global perspective. American Institute for Cancer Research/World Cancer Research Fund, American Institute for Cancer Research, 1997." *Nutrition* 1999 Jun; 15(6):523-6.

Goodman, M.T., Wilkens, L.R., Hankin, J.H., Lyu, L.C., Wu, A.H., Kolonel, L.N. "Association of soy and fiber consumption with the risk of endometrial cancer." *Am. J. Epidemiol.* Aug 15; 146(4):294–306.

Himmelstein, D.U., Thorne, D., Warren, E., Woolhandler, S. "Medical bankruptcy in the United States, 2007: results of a national study." *Am J Med.* 2009 Aug; 122(8):741-6.

Integrated Benefits Institute. www.idiweb.org.

Itoh, H., Noda, H., Amano, H., Zhuaug, C., Mizuno, T., Ito, H. "Antitumor activity and immunological properties of marine algal polysaccharides, especially fucoidan, prepared from Sargassum thunbergii of Phaeophyceae." *Anticancer Res.* 1993 Nov–Dec; 13(6A):2045–52.

Keys, A., Taylor, H.L., Blackburn, H., Brozek, J., Anderson, J.T., Simonson, E. "Coronary Heart Disease among Minnesota Business and Professional Men Followed Fifteen Years." *Circulation* 1963 Sep; 28:381–395.

Kolata, Gina. "A Growing Disenchantment with October 'Pinkification.'" *New York Times* October 30, 2015.

Kushi, L.H., Cunningham, J.E., Hebert, J.R., et al. "The Macrobiotic Diet in Cancer." The *Journal of Nutrition*, Volume 131, Issue 11, November 2001, Pages 3056S–3064S.

Lazarou, J., Pomeranz, B.H., Corey, P.N. "Incidence of adverse drug reactions in hospitalized patients: a meta-analysis of prospective studies." *JAMA* 1998 Apr 15; 279(15):1200–5.

Libby, P. "Inflammation and cardiovascular disease mechanisms." *Am J Clin Nutr.* 2006 Feb; 83(2):456S-460S.

Marcos, A., Nova, E., Montero, A. "Changes in the immune system are conditioned by nutrition." *European Journal of Clinical Nutrition* 2003 Sep; 57 Suppl 1:S66-9.

McDougall, John A. And Mary. The *Starch Solution*. New York: Rodale, 2013.

National Institute for Health and Care Excellence. www.nice.org.uk.

NIH National Cancer Institute. "The Genetics of Cancer." www.cancer.gov/about-cancer/causes-prevention/genetics.

Nishino, H. "Cancer prevention by carotenoids." *Mutat. Res.* 1998 Jun 18; 402(1-2):159-63.

Okuzumi, J., Nishino, H., Murakoshi, M., Iwashima, A., Tanaka, Y., Yamane, T., Fujita, Y., Takahashi, T. "Inhibitory effects of fucoxanthin, a natural carotenoid, on N-myc expression and cell cycle progression in human malignant tumor cells." *Cancer Lett* 1990 Nov 19; 55(1):75–81.

Ornish, D. *Dr. Dean Ornish's Program for Reversing Heart Disease*. New York: Random House, 1990.

Ornish, D.M., Gotto, A.M., Miller, R.R., et al. "Effects of a vegetarian diet and selected yoga techniques in the treatment of coronary heart disease." *Clinical Research* 1979; 27:720A.

Slavin, J.L. "Mechanisms for the impact of whole grain foods on cancer risk." *J Am Coll Nutr*. 2000 Jun; 19(3 Suppl):300S-307S.

Teas, J., Harbison, M.L., Gelman, R.S. "Dietary seaweed [laminaria] and mammary carcinogenesis in rats." *Cancer Res*. 1984 Jul; 44(7):2758-61.

Wellen, K.E., Hotamisligil, G.S. "Inflammation, stress and diabetes." *J Clin Invest*. 2005 May 2; 115(5): 1111–1119.

Yamamoto, I., Maruyama, H., Moriguchi, M. "The effect of dietary seaweeds on 7,12-dimethyl-benz[a]anthracene-induced mammary tumorigenesis in rats." *Cancer Lett* 1987 May; 35(2):109-18.

Chapter 6

Blumenthal, D.M., Gold, M.S. "Neurobiology of Food Addiction." *Current Opinion Clinical Nutritional Metabolism Care* 2010 Jul;13(4):359-65.

Dantzer, R., et al. "From inflammation to sickness and depression: when the immune system subjugates the brain." *National Review of Neuroscience* 2008 Jan; 9(1):46–56.

Lamport, D. "Flavonoids and brain health: Does consuming flavonoid-rich foods benefit cognitive function?" Nutrition and Health Group, School of Psychology and Clinical Language Sciences, University of Reading. https://docplayer.net/50496322-Flavonoids-and-brain-health-does-consuming-flavonoid-rich-foods-benefit-cogni-tive-function.html.

Spencer, J.P. "The impact of flavonoids on memory: physiological and molecular considerations." *Chem Soc Rev*. 2009 Apr; 38(4):1152-61.

Tara, W. *Natural Body Natural Mind*. Bloomington, IN: Xlibris Corp., 2008.

Wenk, G. *Your Brain on Food: How Chemicals Control Your Thoughts and Feelings*. Oxford, UK: Oxford University Press, 2010.

Witherly, S. *Why Humans Like Junk Food*. Bloomington, IN: iUniverse Inc., 2007.

World Health Organization. *WHO Global Report on Traditional and Complementary Medicine 2019*. Geneva: World Health Organization, 2019. www.who.int/tradition-al-complementary-integrative-medicine/WhoGlobalReportOnTraditionalAndCom-plementaryMedicine2019.pdf?ua=1.

Wurtman, Richard J. "Food Components to Enhance Performance: An Evaluation of Potential Performance-Enhancing Food Components for Operational Rations." Institute of Medicine (US) Committee on Military Nutrition Research; Marriott, B.M., editor. Washington (DC): National Academies Press (US), 1994.

Chapter 7

Anderson, E.N., Pearsall, D., Hunn, E., Turner, N., Eds. *Ethnobiology*. Hoboken, NJ: Wiley-Blackwell, 2011.

Anonymous (1895) "Some new ideas. The plants cultivated by aboriginal people and how used in primitive commerce." The *[Daily] Evening Telegraph*, Philadelphia, Thursday, 5 December, Vol. 64, No. 134, p. 2.

Campbell, T.C., Junshi, C. "Diet and chronic degenerative diseases: perspectives from China." *Am J Clin Nutr*. 1994 May; 59(5 Suppl):1153S-1161S.

Dopico, X.C., et al. "Widespread Seasonal Gene Expression Reveals Annual Differences in Human Immunity and Physiology." *Nature Communications* 2015 May 12; 6:7000.

Ford, R.I., Ed. The *Nature and Status of Ethnobotany, 2nd Edition*. Ann Arbor, MI: U of M Museum of Anthro Archaeology, 1994.

Goldman, I.L., Kader, A.A., Heintz, C. "Influence of production, handling, and storage on phytonutrient content of food." *Nutr Rev*. 1999 Sep; 57(9 Pt 2):S46-52.

Harari, Y.N. Sapiens: A Brief History of Humankind. London, UK: Vintage Books, 2014.

Ho, E., Domann, F. *Nutrition and Epigenetics*. Boca Raton, FL: CRC Press, 2015.

May, R.M. "Ecological Science and Tomorrow's World." *Philos Trans R Soc Lond B Biol Sci*. 2010 Jan 12; 365(1537):41–47.

Raven, P.H., Evert, R.F., Eichhorn, S.E. *Biology of Plants, 7th Ed*. New York: W.H. Freeman, 2005.

Ryan, R.M. et al. "Vitalizing effects of being outdoors and in nature." *Journal of Environmental Psychology* June 2010; 30(2):159–168.

Shah, N.S., Nath, N. "Minimally processed fruits and vegetables - Freshness with convenience." *J Food Sci Tech*. 2006 Nov; 43(6): 561–570.

Singh, Amrit Pal. The *Lost Glory of Folk Medicine*. Surrey, UK: Emedia Science Ltd., 2002.

Chapter 8

Centers for Disease Control and Prevention. National Center for Health Statistics, April 2016. www.cdc.gov/nchs/index.htm.

Common Sense. The *Common Sense Census: Media Use by Tweens and Teens*. San Francisco, CA: Common Sense Media Inc., 2015.

Commoner, B. The *Closing Circle: Nature, Man & Technology*. New York: Random House, Inc., 1971.

Freedman D. S., et al. "The Relation of Overweight to Cardiovascular Risk Factors among Children and Adolescents: the Bogalusa Heart Study." *Pediatrics* 1999 June; 103(6):1175.

Klein, Naomi. *This Changes Everything: Capitalism vs. The Climate*. New York: Simon & Schuster, 2015.

Miller, G.J. "Effects of diet composition on coagulation pathways." The *American Journal of Clinical Nutrition*, Volume 67, Issue 3, March 1998, Pages 542S–545S. https://doi.org/10.1093/ajcn/67.3.542S.

Mullikin, Lindsey J. "Beyond reference pricing: Understanding consumers' encounters with unexpected prices." *Journal of Product & Brand Management* 2003 June; 12(3):140–153.

Natural Marketing Institute. www.nmisolutions.com. March 2, 2015.

Nicholls, S.J., Lundman, P., Harmer, J.A., et al. "Consumption of Saturated Fat Impairs the Anti-Inflammatory Properties of High-Density Lipoproteins and Endothelial Function." *J Am Coll Cardiol*. 2006 Aug 15; 48(4):715-20.

Olshansky, S.J., et al. "A Potential Decline in Life Expectancy in the United States in the 21st Century." *New England Journal of Medicine* 2005 Mar 17; 352(11):1138–45.

Pergams, Oliver R.W., Czech B., Haney J.C., Nyberg D. "Linkage of conservation activity to trends in the U.S. economy." *Conservation Biology* 2004; 18:1617–1623.

Pergams, Oliver R.W., Zaradic, Patricia A. "Evidence for a fundamental and pervasive shift away from nature-based recreation." *Proc Natl Acad Sci USA* 2008 Feb 19; 105(7): 2295–2300.

Ulrich, R.S. "View through a window may influence recovery from surgery." *Science* 1984 Apr 27; 224(4647):420-1.

"United States Organic Foods Market Forecast and Opportunities 2020: Organic food products in the US is projected to cross USD 45 billion in 2015." PR Newswire, Research and Markets, 2015 Mar 18. https://www.prnewswire.com/news-releases/united-states-organic-foods-market-forecast-and-opportunities-2020-organic-food-products-in-the-us-is-projected-to-cross-usd45-billion-in-2015-300052511.html.

United States Department of Agriculture. Scientific Report of the 2015 Dietary Guidelines Advisory Committee. Washington, DC, 2015.

Chapter 9

American Society of Civil Engineers. *Failure to Act: the Economic Impact of Current Investment Trends in Water and Waste Treatment Infrastructure*. Washington, DC: American Society of Civil Engineers, 2016. www.asce.org/failuretoact.

Badgley, C., Moghtader, J., et al. "Organic agriculture and the global food supply." *Renewable Agriculture and Food Systems* 22(2); 86–108.

Bellinger, D.C. "Comparing the population neurodevelopmental burdens associated with children's exposures to environmental chemicals and other risk factors." *Neurotoxicology* 2012 Aug; 33(4):641-3.

Congressional Directive. Agriculture, Rural Development, Food and Drug Administration and Related Agencies Appropriations Act, 2015.

Department of International Development. www.gov.uk.

Diamond, J. *Collapse: How Societies Choose to Fail or Survive*. New York: Penguin Books, 2011.

Fedinik, Kristi Pullen, Wu, M., Olson, E.D. "Threats on Tap: Widespread Violations Highlight Need for Investment in Water Infrastructure and Protections." NRDC. May 2, 2017. www.nrdc.org/resources/threats-tap-widespread-violations-water-infra-structure.

Food and Agriculture Organization of the United Nations, Technical Workshop. *Biodiversity in Sustainable Diets. Rome, 31 May–1 June 2010*. Rome: FAO, 2010.

Friends of the Earth. *What's Feeding Our Food?* December 2008. https://friendsofthee-arth.uk/sites/default/files/downloads/livestock_impacts.pdf.

Grace Communications Foundation. Water Footprint Calculator. www.watercalcu-lator.org.

Green Alliance policy insight, April 2012. "What people really think of the environ-ment." www.green-alliance.org.uk/resources/What%20people%20really%20think.pdf.

Haard, N., Odunfa, S.A., et al. *Fermented Cereals: A Global Perspective*. Fao Agricultural Services Bulletin No.138. www.fao.org/3/x2184e/x2184e00.htm.

Hoekstra. A.Y., Ed. *Virtual Water Trade. Proceedings of the International Expert Meeting on Virtual Water Trade*. IHE Delft, the Netherlands, 12–13 December 2002. Research Report Series No.12, February, 2003.

Institution of Mechanical Engineers. "Global Food: Waste Not, Want Not." 2 Nov 2013. IMechE. www.imeche.org/policy-and-press/reports/detail/global-food-waste-not-want-not.

Kaldy, M.S. "Protein yield of various crops as related to protein value." Economic Botany April 1972; 26(2):142–144.

Linking Environment and Farming. www.leafuk.org.

Livestock, Environment and Development (LEAD) Initiative. *Livestock's Long Shadow*. Rome: FAO, 2006. www.fao.org/3/a0701e/a0701e00.htm.

Messina, M.J. "Legumes and soybeans: overview of their nutritional profiles and health effects." *Am J Clin Nutr*. 1999 Sep; 70(3 Suppl):439S-450S.

Nellemann, C., Miles, L., Kaltenborn, B. P., Virtue, M., and Ahlenius, H., Eds. *The Last Stand of the Orangutan*. United Nations Environment Programme, 2007.

NOAA Headquarters. "NOAA: Gulf of Mexico 'dead zone' predictions feature uncertainty." Phys.org, June 21, 2012. https://phys.org/news/2012-06-noaa-gulf-mexico-dead-zone.html.

Pesticide Action Network International. "PAN Listing of Highly Hazardous Pesti-cides, December 2016." www.panna.org/sites/default/files/PAN_HHP_List%20 2016.pdf.

Schinasi, L., Leon, M.E. "Non-Hodgkin lymphoma and occupational exposure to agricultural pesticide chemical groups and active ingredients: a systematic review and meta-analysis." *International Journal of Environmental Research and Public Health* 2014 Apr 23; 11(4): 4449-527.

September 2014 EWG Report / April 2015 update. www.ewg.org.

Smithsonian, National Museum of Natural History, Ocean Portal. "Ocean Acidification."

https://ocean.si.edu/ocean-life/invertebrates/ocean-acidification.

The Water Footprint Network. http://waterfootprint.org.

U.S. Department of Veterans Affairs. *Agent Orange Benefits Report.* 1997.

United States Environmental Protection Agency. "Ground Water and Drinking Water. Basic Information on Lead in Drinking Water." www.epa.gov/ground-water-and-drinking-water/basic-information-about-lead-drinking-water.

White, Kate. "Monsanto vows $93M to Nitro residents." *Charleston Gazette-Mail* February 24, 2012. https://www.wvgazettemail.com/news/special_reports/monsanto-vows-m-to-nitro-residents/article_a50fe819-fe31-5d1a-a743-c7cd0ea0b1c4.html.

World Business Council for Sustainable Development. "Water: Facts and trends." www.wbcsd.org/Programs/Food-Land-Water/Water/Resources/Water-Facts-and-trends.

World Health Organization. "Dioxins and their effects on human health." WHO Fact sheet N°225, updated 4 October 2016. https://www.who.int/news-room/fact-sheets/detail/dioxins-and-their-effects-on-human-health.

Chapter 10

"27 Mexican Celery Workers Die as Train Hits Bus in California." *New York Times,* 18 September 1963.

"Bracero Train-Truck Crash Toll Reaches 31." *Monterey Peninsula Herald,* 20 September 1963.

"Crash Kills 27: Train Smashes Makeshift Bus." *Los Angeles Times,* 18 September 1963.

"Playing Politics with Tragedy." *Salinas Californian,* 19 September 1963.

American Academy of Child and Adolescent Psychiatry. "Obesity in Children and Teens." *Facts for Families* No.79; Apr 2016. www.aacap.org/aacap/families_and_youth/facts_for_families/fff-guide/obesity-in-children-and-teens-079.aspx.

Bohme, S. "People v. Dole." *Boston Review* July 14, 2014. http://bostonreview.net/world/susanna-bohme-dole-banana-workers-pesticide-nicaragua.

Campbell, D. "Taco's tomato pickers on slave wages." The *Guardian* 16 Mar 2003. www.theguardian.com/world/2003/mar/17/usa.duncancampbell.

Coalition of Immokalee Workers. "Tag: Slavery." https://ciw-online.org/blog/tag/slavery.

De Las Casas, B. "A Short Account of the Destruction of the Indies." New York: Penguin Classics, 1992.

Dodson, H. *Jubilee: the Emergence of African-American Culture.* Washington, DC: National Geographic Books, 2003.

Drewnowski. A., Specter, S.E. "Poverty and obesity: the role of energy density and energy costs." *Am J Clin Nutr.* 2004 Jan; 79(1):6-16.

Fitzgerald, A.J., Kalof, L., Dietz, T. "Slaughterhouses and Increased Crime Rates—An Empirical Analysis of the Spillover from "The Jungle" into the Surrounding Community." *Organization & Environment* June 2, 2009; 22(2):158-184.

Freeman, A. "Fast Food: Oppression through Poor Nutrition." *California Law Review* Dec 31, 2007; 95(6).

Gravenor, M., Ed. "Objectively Measured Physical Activity and Fat Mass in Children: A Bias-Adjusted Meta-Analysis of Prospective Studies." *PLoS One* 2011; 6(2): e17205.

Hodal, K., Kelly, C., Lawrence, F. "Revealed: Asian slave labour producing prawns for supermarkets in US, UK." The *Guardian,* June 10, 2014. www.theguardian.com/global-development/2014/jun/10/supermarket-prawns-thailand-produced-slave-labour.

International Scientific Symposium on Biodiversity and Sustainable Diets United Against Hunger, Final Document, November 2010. United Nations Food and Agriculture Organization, FAO Rome.

Interstate Commerce Commission, Railroad Accident Investigation, Ex Parte No. 237, Southern Pacific Company, Chualar, California, September 17, 1963. 260.

Kandel, William. "Recent Trends in Rural-based Meat Processing." Economic Research Service, U.S. Department of Agriculture citing Bureau of Labor statistic.

Kanji, N. "Corporate Responsibility and Women's Employment: the Cashew Nut Case." *International Institute for Environment and Development* March 2004; no.2.

Lincoln, Jennifer. "Commercial Fishing Safety Research." *National Institute for Occupational Safety and Health* April 29, 2008.

Lubin, G., Badkar, M. "15 Facts About McDonald's That Will Blow Your Mind." *Business Insider* November 25, 2011. www.businessinsider.com/facts-about-mcdonalds-blow-your-mind-2011-11.

Mandeel, E.W. "The Bracero Program 1942-1964." *American International Journal of Contemporary Research* January 2014; 4(1).

McWilliams, J. "PTSD in the Slaughterhouse." The *Texas Observer,* February 7, 2012. www.texasobserver.org/ptsd-in-the-slaughterhouse.

Moore, Truman E. The *Slaves We Rent.* New York: Random House, 1965.

National Statistics. "Households below Average Income." London, UK: Department for Work and Pensions, 2005.

Nestle, M. *Soda Politics: Taking on Big Soda (and Winning).* Oxford, UK: Oxford University Press, 2015.

O'Connor, A. "Coca-Cola Funds Scientists Who Shift the Blame for Obesity Away From Bad Diets." *New York Times,* August 9, 2015. https://well.blogs.nytimes.com/2015/08/09/coca-cola-funds-scientists-who-shift-blame-for-obesity-away-from-bad-diets.

Orwell, G. The *Road to Wigan Pier*. New York: Penguin Classics, 1937.

Pacific Lutheran University. *Bananas: Environmental Impacts of Banana Growing*. https://community.plu.edu/~bananas/environmental/home.html.

Palmunen, A. "Learning from the mistakes of the past: an analysis of past and current temporary worker policies and their implications for a twenty-first century guest worker program." *Kennedy School Review* 2005; 6:47.

Rodriguez, J.P. *Historical Encyclopedia of World Slavery*. Santa Barbara, CA: ABC-CLIO, 1997.

Royle, T. *Working for McDonald's in Europe: the Unequal Struggle*. New York: Routledge, 2004.

Schlosser, E. "The Chain Never Stops." *Mother Jones*. July/Aug 2001. www.motherjones.com/politics/2001/07/dangerous-meatpacking-jobs-eric-schlosser.

Skinner, B. "Indonesia's Palm Oil Industry Rife With Human-Rights Abuses." *Bloomberg Businessweek* July 20, 2013. www.bloomberg.com/news/articles/2013-07-18/indonesias-palm-oil-industry-rife-with-human-rights-abuses

U.S. Government Accountability Office. "Workplace Safety and Health: Safety in the Meat and Poultry Industry, While Improving, Could Be Further Strengthened." GAO-05-96: Jan 12, 2005. Publicly Released: Jan 28, 2005.

Urbina, I. "Forced Labor for Cheap Fish." *New York Times*, July 27, 2015, no.56,940.

Vogel, R.D. "Transient Servitude: the U.S. Guest Worker Program for Exploiting Mexican and Central American Workers." *Monthly Review* Jan 1, 2007. https://monthlyreview.org/2007/01/01/transient-servitude-the-u-s-guest-worker-program-for-exploiting-mexican-and-central-american-workers.

Chapter 11

Davis, M. The *Monster at Our Door*. New York: Holt Paperbacks, 2006.

Grandin, T. The *Effect of Economics on the Welfare of Cattle, Pigs, Sheep, and Poultry*. Department of Animal Sciences, Colorado State University, April 2013. www.grandin.com/welfare/economic.effects.welfare.html.

Dillard, J. "A Slaughterhouse Nightmare: Psychological Harm Suffered by Slaughterhouse Employees and the Possibility of Redress through Legal Reform." *Georgetown Journal on Poverty Law & Policy* 2008; 15(2);391–408.

Francione, G.L., Charlton, A. *Animal Rights: the Abolitionist Approach*. Warsaw, Poland: Exempla Press, 2015.

Ishige, N. The *History and Culture of Japanese Food*. New York: Routledge, 2001.

Lewis, C. S. The *Screwtape Letters*. New York: HarperOne, 2015.

Low, P. The *Cambridge Declaration on Consciousness*. Publicly proclaimed in Cambridge, UK, on July 7, 2012, at the Francis Crick Memorial Conference on Consciousness in Human and non-Human Animals, at Churchill College, University of Cambridge, by Low, Edelman and Koch.

Mark, J. "Toward a Moral Case for Meat Eating." *Sierra* Feb 24, 2017. www.sierraclub.org/sierra/green-life/toward-moral-case-for-meat-eating.

Natural Resources Defense Council. "Facts about Pollution from Livestock Farms." http://ogoapes.weebly.com/uploads/3/2/3/9/3239894/water_pollution_from_livestock_farms.pdf.

Ohsawa, G. The *Book of Judgement: Philosophy of Macrobiotics*. Oroville, CA: George Oshawa Macrobiotic Foundation,1980.

Porphyry; Taylor, T., Ed. *Porphyry on Abstinence from Animal Food*. London, UK: Centaur Press, 1965.

Sinclair, U. The *Jungle*. Mineola, NY: Dover Publications, 2001.

Slow Food. "A Talk with Peter Singer." 27 Apr 2009. www.slowfood.com/a-talk-with-peter-singer.

Smith, K.L., Hillerton, J.E., Harmon, R.J. *Guidelines on normal and abnormal raw milk based on somatic cell counts and signs of clinical mastitis*. Madison, WI: NMC, Inc., 2001.

Spencer, C. The *Heretic's Feast: A History of Vegetarianism*. Lebanon, NH: University Press of New England, 1995.

Sterbenz, C. "7 Reasons Why I Refuse to Stop Eating Meat." *Business Insider* Sept. 30, 2013. www.businessinsider.com/reasons-to-eat-meat-2013-9.

Taylor, L.H., Latham, S.M., Woolhouse, M.E. "Risk factors for human disease emergence." *Philos Trans R Soc Lond B Biol Sci*. 2001 Jul 29; 356(1411):983-9.

The Young and Hungry. "Interview with Jonathan Safran Foer." May 3, 2009. https://web.archive.org/web/20090509003808/http://www.theyoungandhungry.com/1241412745/interview-with-jonathan-safran-foer.

Chapter 12

Allen, L.H. "How common is vitamin B-12 deficiency?" Am J Clin Nutr. 2009 Feb; 89(2):693S-6S.

Bjerregaard, P., Young, T.K., Hegele, R.A. "Low incidence of cardiovascular disease among the Inuit—what is the evidence?" *Atherosclerosis* 2003 Feb; 166(2):351-7.

Bozian, R.C., Ferguson, J.L., Heyssel, R.M., Meneely, G.R., Darby, W.J. "Evidence concerning the human requirement for vitamin B12. Use of the whole body counter for determination of absorption of vitamin B12. *Am J Clin Nutr*. 1963 Feb; 12:117-29.

Genetherapy.me. "Omega-3 fatty acids. University of Maryland Medical Center." www.genetherapy.me/inflammation/omega-3-fatty-acids-university-of-maryland-medical-center.php.

Mbalilaki, J.A., Masesa, Z., Stromme, S.B., et al. "Daily energy expenditure and cardiovascular risk in Masai, rural, and urban Bantu Tanzanians." *British Journal of Sports Medicine*, 2010 Feb; 44(2):121-6.

Simopoulos, A.P. "Evolutionary aspects of diet: the omega-6/omega-3 ratio and the brain. *Molecular Neurobiology* 2011 Oct; 44(2):203–15.

USDA Economic Research Service. Profiling Food Consumption in America, 2000.

Vogel, R.A., et al. "The postprandial effect of components of the Mediterranean diet on endothelial function." *J Am Coll Cardiol*. 2000 Nov 1; 36(5):1455-60.

Watanabe, F., Takenaka, S., Katsura, H., Masumder, S.A., Abe, K., Tamura, Y., Nakano, Y. "Dried green and purple lavers (Nori) contain substantial amounts of biologically active vitamin B(12) but less of dietary iodine relative to other edible seaweeds." *J Agric Food Chem*. 1999 Jun; 47(6):2341-3.

Chapter 13

Barrett, Julia R. "The Science of Soy: What Do We Really Know?" *Environ Health Perspect*. 2006 Jun; 114(6): A352–A358.

Caan, B.J., Natarajan, L., et al. "Soy food consumption and breast cancer prognosis." *Cancer Epidemiol Biomarkers Prev*. 2011 May; 20(5):854-8.

Chandrasekara, A., Shahidi, F. "Content of insoluble bound phenolics in millets and their contribution to antioxidant capacity." *J Agric Food Chem*. 2010 Jun 9;58(11):6706-14.

Davis, J. et al. "Environmental impact of four meals with different protein sources: Case studies in Spain and Sweden." *Food Research International* August 2010; 43(7):1874–1884.

Fernandez, Maria Luz; West, Kristy L. "Mechanisms by which Dietary Fatty Acids Modulate Plasma Lipids." The *Journal of Nutrition* September 2005; 135(9):2075–2078.

Food Allergy Research & Education. www.foodallergy.org.

Fraser, G.E., Sabaté, J., Beeson, W.L., Strahan, T.M. "A possible protective effect of nut consumption on risk of coronary heart disease. The Adventist Health Study." *Arch Intern Med*. 1992 Jul; 152(7):1416-24.

Holdt, S. Løvstad; Kraan, S. "Bioactive Compounds in Seaweed: Functional Food Applications and Legislation." *Journal of Applied Psychology* 2011; 23(3):543–597.

Kurozawa, Y. et al. "Dietary habits and risk of death due to hepatocellular carcinoma in a large-scale cohort study in Japan. Univariate analysis of JACC study data." *Kurume Medical Journal* 2004; 51(2):141–9.

Lee, S.H., et al. "Millet consumption decreased serum concentration of triglyceride and C-reactive protein but not oxidative status in hyperlipidemic rats." *Nutrition Research* 2010 Apr; 30(4):290–6.

Setchell, K. "Exposure of infants to phyto-oestrogens from soy-based infant formula." *Lancet* 1997 July 5; 350(9070):23-7.

Sharp, G.B., et al. "Relationship of hepatocellular carcinoma to soy food consumption: a cohort-based, case-control study in Japan." *International Journal of Cancer* 2005 Jun 10; 115(2):290–5.

Steinmetz, K.A., Potter, J.D. "Vegetables, Fruit, and Cancer Prevention." *Journal of the Academy of Nutrition and Dietetics* October 1996; 96(10):1027–1039.

Teas, J. "The dietary intake of Laminaria, a brown seaweed, and breast cancer prevention." *Nutr Cancer*. 1983; 4(3):217-22.

Teixeira, S.R., et al. "Isolated Soy Protein Consumption Reduces Urinary Albumin Excretion and Improves the Serum Lipid Profile in Men with Type 2 Diabetes Mellitus and Nephropathy." *J Nutr*. 2004 Aug; 134(8):1874-80.

UC Davis Integrative Medicine. *Integrative Medicine Bulletin*. August 3, 2016. https://ucdintegrativemedicine.com.

Watanabe, H. "Beneficial Biological Effects of Miso with Reference to Radiation Injury, Cancer, and Hypertension." *J Toxicol Pathol*. 2013 Jun; 26(2): 91–103.

Watson-Tara, M. *Go Vegan*. West Sussex, UK: Lotus Publishing, 2019.

Yamamota, S. et al. "Soy, Isoflavones, and Breast Cancer Risk in Japan." *Journal of the National Cancer Institute* 2003 Jun 18; 95(12):906-13.

Chapter 14

"Arrhenius, Svante August" in *Chamber's Encyclopedia, Vol. 1*. London, UK: George Newnes, 1961.

Caiazzo, F. et al. "Air pollution and early deaths in the United States. Part 1: Quantifying the impact of major sectors in 2005." *Atmospheric Environment* 2013 Nov; 79:198–208.

Center on Addiction. "The Importance of Family Dinners VIII." Sept. 2012. www.centeronaddiction.org/addiction-research/reports/importance-of-family-dinners-2012.

Chowdhury, R., Warnakula, S., Kunutsor, S., et al. "Association of dietary, circulating, and supplement fatty acids with coronary risk." *Ann Intern Med* 2014; 160(6):398–406.

Cook, J., et al. "Consensus on consensus: a synthesis of consensus estimates on human-caused global warming." *Environmental Research Letters* 13 April 2016; 11(4).

de Goede, J., Geleijnse, J.M., Boer, J.M., Kromhout, D., Verschuren, W.M. "Linoleic acid intake, plasma cholesterol and 10-year incidence of CHD in 20,000 middle-aged men and women in the Netherlands." *Br J Nutr* 2011 Aug; 107(7):1070–6.

Harvard T. H. Chan School of Public Health. "New Dietary Guidelines remove restriction on total fat and set limit for added sugars but censor conclusions of the scientific advisory committee." The *Nutrition Source* January 7, 2016. www.hsph.harvard.edu/nutritionsource/2016/01/07/new-dietary-guidelines-remove-restriction-on-total-fat-and-set-limit-for-added-sugars-but-censor-conclusions.

Iraq Body Count. www.iraqbodycount.org. July 24, 2012.

Karkanas, P., Shahack-Gross, R., Ayalon, A., et al. "Evidence for habitual use of fire at the end of the Lower Paleolithic: site formation process at Qesem Cave, Israel" *Journal of Human Evolution* 2007 Aug; 53(2):197–212.

Laaksonen, D.E., Nyyssonen, K., Niskanen, L., Rissanen, T.H., Salonen, J.T. "Prediction of cardiovascular mortality in middle-aged men by dietary and serum linoleic and polyunsaturated fatty acids." *Arch Intern Med*. 2005 Jan 24; 165:193–199.

Oh, K., Hu, F.B., Manson, J.E., Stampfer, M.J., Willett, W.C. "Dietary fat intake and risk of coronary heart disease in women: 20 years of follow-up of the Nurses' Health Study." *Am J Epidemiol.* 2005 Apr 1;161(7):672–9.

Organisation for Economic Co-operation and Development. "OECD 2014 *PISA in Focus* – 2014/01 (January)." www.oecd.org/pisa/pisaproducts/pisainfocus/PISA-in-Focus-n35-(eng)-FINAL.pdf.

Plumer, B. "Nine facts about terrorism in the United States since 9/11" *Washington Post* September 11, 2013.

United Nations Food and Agriculture Organization, FAO Newsroom. "Livestock a Major Threat to the Environment." 29 Nov 2006. www.fao.org/newsroom/en/news/2006/1000448/index.html.

US Department of Agriculture, Economic Research Service. Food CPI, Prices and Expenditures: Sales of Meals and Snacks Away from Home by Type of Outlet, 1929–2007.

Wang, Y. "Epidemiology of Childhood Obesity—Methodological Aspects and Guidelines: What's New?" *Int J Obes Relat Metab Disord.* 2004 Nov; 28 Suppl 3:S21–8.

Watson-Tara, M. *Go Vegan.* West Sussex, UK: Lotus Publishing, 2019.

About the Author

Bill Tara has been an active and long-time advocate for natural health care. He has served as a faculty member for the Kiental Institute in Switzerland and the Naropa University in Boulder, Colorado and is a senior teacher at the International Macrobiotic Institute of Portugal. He was Chairman of the European Macrobiotic Assembly for four years and served as Chairman of the North American Macrobiotic Congress for two years. He was also Director of Natural Health Care at the famous SHA Wellness Clinic in Spain.

Tara has been a health counselor, teacher, author, entrepreneur, and creator of health education centers in Europe and North America. His innovative and creative teaching of traditional approaches to health, healing, and personal development have taken him to over twenty countries as a seminar leader. He has appeared on a variety of radio and television shows in England, America, and Australia, speaking on dietary policy and human ecology. In 2019 he was awarded the Kushi Peace Prize for his over 50 years of service for health, peace, and sustainability.

He founded the Community Health Foundation in London, England, which was the largest natural health education center in the world. He was also the co-founder of the Kushi Institute and served as Executive Director of the institute's programs in both London and Boston. Together with his wife, Marlene Watson-Tara, he teaches workshops and intensive training in macrobiotics, vegan nutrition, and natural health care.

$\mathcal{I}$ndex

Other Square One Titles of Interest

Your Blood Never Lies

How to Read a Blood Test for a Longer, Healthier Life

James B. LaValle, RPh, CCN

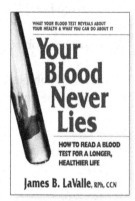

A standard blood test indicates how well the kidneys and liver are functioning, the potential for heart disease, and a host of other vital health markers. Unfortunately, most of us cannot decipher these results ourselves or even formulate the right questions to ask—or we couldn't, until now. *Your Blood Never Lies* clears the mystery surrounding blood test results. In simple language, Dr. LaValle explains all of the information found on these forms, making it understandable and accessible so that you can look at the results yourself and know the significance of each marker.

$16.95 US • 368 pages • 6 x 9-inch paperback • ISBN 978-0-7570-0350-9

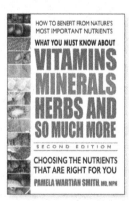

What You Must Know About Vitamins, Minerals, Herbs and So Much More, SECOND EDITION

Choosing the Nutrients That Are Right for You

Pamela Wartian Smith, MD, MPH

Even if you follow a healthful diet, you are probably not getting all the nutrients you need to prevent disease. Why? There are many reasons, ranging from the mineral-depleted soils in which our foods are grown, to medications that rob the body of various vitamins and minerals. Reflecting the latest scientific research, *What You Must Know About Vitamins, Minerals, Herbs and So Much More—Second Edition* explains how you can restore and maintain health through the wise use of nutrients. Whether you are trying to overcome a medical condition or you simply want to preserve good health, this book will guide you in making the best dietary and supplement choices.

$16.95 US • 512 pages • 6 x 9-inch paperback • ISBN 978-0-7570-0471-1

The Acid-Alkaline Food Guide

SECOND EDITION

A Quick Reference to Foods &
Their Effect on pH Levels

Susan E. Brown, PhD, and Larry Trivieri, Jr.

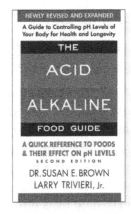

The importance of acid-alkaline balance to good health is no secret. *The Acid-Alkaline Food Guide* was designed as an easy-to-follow guide to the most common foods that influence your body's pH level. Now in its second edition, this bestseller has been expanded to include many more domestic and international foods. Updated information also explores (and refutes) the myths about pH balance and diet, and guides you to supplements that can help you achieve a pH level that supports greater well-being.

$8.95 US • 224 pages • 4 x 7-inch paperback • ISBN 978-0-7570-0393-6

Glycemic Index Food Guide

For Weight Loss, Cardiovascular Health, Diabetic Management, and Maximum Energy

Dr. Shari Lieberman

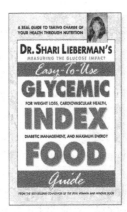

By indicating how quickly a given food triggers a rise in blood sugar, the glycemic index (GI) enables you to choose foods that can help you manage a variety of conditions and improve your overall health. This easy-to-use guide teaches you about the GI and how to use it. It provides both the glycemic index and the glycemic load for hundreds of foods and beverages, including raw foods, cooked foods, and many combination and prepared foods. Whether you want to manage your diabetes, lose weight, increase your heart health, or simply enhance your well-being, the *Glycemic Index Food Guide* is the best place to start.

$7.95 US • 160 pages • 4 x 7-inch paperback • ISBN 978-0-7570-0245-8

Suicide by Sugar

A Startling Look at Our #1 National Addiction

Nancy Appleton, PhD, and G.N. Jacobs

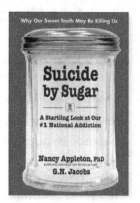

More than three decades ago, Nancy Appleton's *Lick the Sugar Habit* exposed the health dangers of America's high-sugar diet. Now, in *Suicide by Sugar,* Appleton, along with journalist G.N. Jacobs, presents a broader view of the problems caused by our favorite ingredient. The authors offer startling facts linking a range of disorders—from dementia and hypoglycemia to obesity and cancer—to our growing addiction to sugar. Rounding out the book, they present a sound diet plan that leads the way to good health, along with a number of recipes for sweet, easy-to-prepare, delectable dishes—all made without sugar or fruit.

$15.95 US • 192 pages • 6 x 9-inch paperback • ISBN 978-0-7570-0306-6

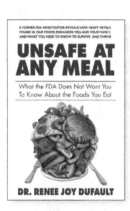

Unsafe at Any Meal

What the FDA Does Not Want You to Know About the Foods You Eat

Dr. Renee Joy Dufault

Each year, Americans consume hundreds of food products that contain dangerous compounds, including heavy metals, pesticides, and harmful additives. Why haven't we heard about this? In *Unsafe at Any Meal,* Dr. Renee Dufault, former food investigator for the Food and Drug Administration, provides the startling answers. Dr. Dufault also presents an in-depth look at the toxic substances commonly found in our food supply and explains how they affect our genes, our health, and the surrounding environment. Backed by research and first-hand experience, Dr. Dufault reveals how the FDA has failed us, and outlines how you can protect yourself and your family by knowing which foods to avoid.

$16.95 US • 240 pages • 6 x 9-inch paperback • ISBN 978-0-7570-0436-0

Greens and Grains on the Deep Blue Sea Cookbook

Fabulous Vegetarian Cuisine from the Holistic Holiday at Sea Cruises

Sandy Pukel and Mark Hanna

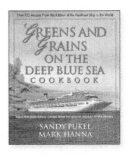

Come aboard one of America's premier health cruises. Too busy to get away? No problem. You can still enjoy its gourmet cuisine, thanks to *Greens and Grains on the Deep Blue Sea Cookbook*—a titanic collection of the most popular vegetarian dishes served aboard the Holistic Holiday at Sea cruises. Written by natural foods expert Sandy Pukel and master chef Mark Hanna, this book provides an innovative selection of over 120 taste-tempting appetizers, soups, salads, entrées, side dishes, and desserts—all as delicious as they are nutritious.

$16.95 US • 160 pages • 7.5 x 9-inch paperback • ISBN 978-0-7570-0287-8

The World Goes Raw Cookbook

An International Collection of Raw Vegetarian Recipes

Lisa Mann

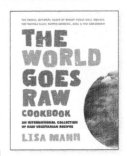

Although raw food can be delicious and improve your well-being, raw cuisine cookbooks have always offered little variety—until now. In this book, chef Lisa Mann provides a fresh approach to (un)cooking. After guiding you in stocking your kitchen with the tools and ingredients that make it easy to prepare raw meals, Lisa presents a variety of taste-tempting international dishes highlighting the cuisines of Italy, Mexico, Asia, South America, the Caribbean, and the Middle East.

$16.95 US • 176 pages • 7.5 x 9-inch paperback • ISBN 978-0-7570-0320-2

Vicki's Vegan Kitchen

Eating with Sanity, Compassion & Taste

Vicki Chelf

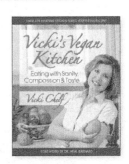

Vegan dishes are healthy and delicious, yet many people are daunted by the idea of preparing meals that contain no animal products. Vicki Chelf presents a comprehensive cookbook designed to take the mystery out of meatless meals. The book begins with an overview of the vegan diet and chapters on kitchen staples, cooking methods, and food preparation. Over 375 of Vicki's favorite recipes follow.

$17.95 US • 320 pages • 7.5 x 9-inch paperback • ISBN 978-0-7570-0251-9

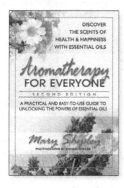

Aromatherapy for Everyone
SECOND EDITION

Discover the Scents of Health and Happiness with Essential Oils

P.J. Pierson and Mary Shipley

It's a well-known fact that essential oils can relax, stimulate, and even heal, but how do you know which ones to use? *Aromatherapy for Everyone* provides easy-to-understand information on how to choose and use the essential oils that are right for you.

$12.95 US • 184 pages • 6 x 9-inch paperback • ISBN 978-0-7570-0473-5

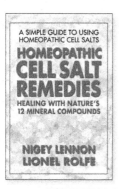

Homeopathic Cell Salt Remedies

Healing with Nature's 12 Mineral Compounds

Nigey Lennon and Lionel Rolfe

Homeopathic Cell Salt Remedies is a simple, comprehensive guide to healing with mineral compounds called cell salts. The book provides full descriptions of the twelve cell salts and discusses how they can be used to treat common conditions.

$12.95 US • 160 pages • 6 x 9-inch paperback • ISBN 978-0-7570-0250-2

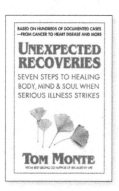

Unexpected Recoveries

Seven Steps to Healing Body, Mind, and Soul
When Serious Illness Strikes

Tom Monte

Unexpected Recoveries is an inspiring guide for those who suffer from life-threatening health conditions. Readers are provided with a flexible seven-step program to help them on their journey of healing. Mental attitude, lifestyle, diet, and exercise are discussed in an easy-to-read manner.

$17.95 US • 256 pages • 6 x 9-inch paperback • ISBN 978-0-7570-0400-1

**For more information on our books,
visit our website at www.squareonepublishers.com**
